DIFFICULT AIRWAY
MANAGEMENT
Case Studies

Ambreen Yasin
Carl Groves
Aleksandra Reszka
Cyprian Mendonca

tfm Publishing Limited, Castle Hill Barns, Harley, Shrewsbury, SY5 6LX, UK
Tel: +44 (0)1952 510061; Fax: +44 (0)1952 510192
E-mail: info@tfmpublishing.com; Web site: www.tfmpublishing.com

Editing: Dr. Christine Graham PhD
Editing, design & typesetting: Nikki Bramhill BSc (Hons), Dip Law
Cover photo: © iStock.com
Credit: ChaNaWiT; stock illustration ID: 471759414

First edition:	© September 2023
Paperback	ISBN: 978-1-913755-36-2
E-book editions:	© January 2024
ePub	ISBN: 978-1-913755-37-9
Mobi	ISBN: 978-1-913755-38-6
Web pdf	ISBN: 978-1-913755-39-3

Printed by L&C PRINTING GROUP, Tadeusza Romanowicza 11, 30-702 Kraków, Poland
Tel: +48 690 565 600; E-mail: office@lcprinting.eu; Web site: www.lcprinting.eu

Contents

Preface

Every student has their own learning style. In medicine, in the early part of a doctor's career, most knowledge is acquired through reading books and attending regular teaching sessions. Following graduation, every doctor has a responsibility for lifelong learning. Reflective learning based on one's own clinical practice becomes the pillar of learning. Clinical cases form a rich resource for reflective learning. Reflection leads to a specific, measurable, achievable and time-bound action plan that enhances learning.

The *Difficult Airway Management — Case Studies* book aims to take the reader through the practicalities of difficult airway management using clinical scenarios to frame the important airway skills required of airway practitioners. Each topic is presented using a real-life clinical case experienced, followed by specific learning points that would improve patient safety in airway management. Some of the cases described in this book predate the availability of current guidelines and equipment. Therefore, they were managed with the existing knowledge and equipment at that time. In the past, a Macintosh laryngoscope, McCoy laryngoscope and fibreoptic bronchoscope were the three devices available for laryngoscopy and tracheal intubation. Over the last two decades, with advancing technology, a series of guidelines and increased knowledge on human factors have enabled us to manage a patient's airway more safely.

This book offers the authors' view on how these situations could be managed if they were to arise again. Reflecting upon these cases has given us an opportunity to see how we could mitigate any complications and how technological advances and recent information may have changed our clinical approach of these cases from the outset. By combining the current evidence base in difficult airway management, this book aims to provide the reader with the basic tools and knowledge to adapt to their personal practice toward safe airway management. We hope this book will prove a valuable resource for all clinicians involved in airway management.

Acknowledgements

We are grateful to colleagues in our department for sharing the case scenarios for the purpose of teaching and learning. We thank Mr Jason McAllister, Graphic Designer, University Hospitals Coventry & Warwickshire NHS Trust for his help with the illustrations. We are indebted to Nikki Bramhill, Director of tfm publishing, and Christine Graham, Editor for tfm publishing, for critically reviewing the manuscript. Sincere thanks go to all the patients who agreed to participate in our airway studies.

Abbreviations

AEC	Airway exchange catheter
AIC	Aintree intubation catheter
APL	Adjustable pressure-limiting
ATI	Awake tracheal intubation
AWS	Airway Scope
BAPM	British Association of Perinatal Medicine
BMI	Body mass index
BP	Blood pressure
BURP	Backward, upward, rightward pressure
Ce	Effect site concentration
CPAP	Continuous positive airway pressure
CT	Computed tomography
CXR	Chest X-ray
DAS	Difficult Airway Society
ECG	Electrocardiogram
ENT	Ear, nose and throat
$ETCO_2$	End-tidal carbon dioxide
ETT	Endotracheal tube
FONA	Front-of-neck access
GCS	Glasgow Coma Scale
HDU	High dependency unit
HELP	Head-elevated laryngoscopy position
HME	Heat and moisture exchange
HR	Heart rate
ICU	Intensive care unit
ILMA	Intubating laryngeal mask airway
LAST	Local anaesthetic systemic toxicity
LMA	Laryngeal mask airway
MDT	Multidisciplinary team
MRI	Magnetic resonance imaging
NAP	National Audit Project

NCEPOD	National Confidential Enquiry into Patient Outcome and Death
NIBP	Non-invasive blood pressure
NTSP	National Tracheostomy Safety Project
ODP	Operating department practitioner
OSA	Obstructive sleep apnoea
PEG	Percutaneous endoscopic gastrostomy
QRH	Quick Reference Handbook
SAD	Supraglottic airway device
SALAD	Suction-Assisted Laryngoscopy and Decontamination
TCI	Target-controlled infusion
TSH	Thyroid stimulating hormone
VAFI	Video-assisted fibreoptic intubation
VL	Videolaryngoscope

Case scenario 1

Introduction

A 56-year-old man presented to the emergency department with a 3-day history of symptoms consistent with acute tonsillitis. He had not received any treatment before admission. After developing difficulties in breathing, in addition to the sore throat, hoarse voice and painful swallowing, he chose to seek medical advice.

Past medical history

Other than a high body mass index of $39kg/m^2$, there was no other significant past medical history.

Clinical examination

On examination, he appeared breathless with no evidence of stridor. Erythema was visible on the right side of the neck.

His observations on admission showed:

- A respiratory rate of 24 breaths/minute.
- Oxygen saturation of 92% in air.
- He was pyrexial.
- Heart rate was 130 beats/minute.
- Blood pressure was maintained at 130/80mmHg.

On auscultation of the chest, there were no abnormal findings. An enlarged tonsil with a purulent exudate was noted when the throat was examined.

The duty anaesthetist attended the patient and conducted an airway assessment that found:

- Mallampati score 2.
- Class B jaw protrusion.
- Normal thyromental distance.
- The patient had a full beard.

Investigations

There were no further investigation results available.

A diagnosis of a parapharyngeal abscess was made, and emergency surgical drainage was planned. Oxygen was administered via a face mask at 15L/minute.

How this case was managed

The patient was transferred to the operating theatre using standard monitoring of pulse oximetry, an electrocardiogram (ECG) and non-invasive blood pressure (NIBP). The team was assembled for a team briefing and consisted of a consultant anaesthetist, a senior trainee in anaesthesia and a consultant ear, nose and throat (ENT) surgeon.

It was noted that clinically the patient was breathless, appeared tired and was not able to receive and retain any further information by this point.

Intubation strategy

Awake intubation using a fibreoptic scope was judged to be challenging due to the lack of patient cooperation. Therefore, a high-risk general anaesthesia induction was planned. The team members, including theatre staff, were informed about the decision. Plan B was to perform a surgical tracheostomy. It was ensured that the surgeon was scrubbed and ready, and the staff were informed to keep the tracheostomy set ready.

In this case, intravenous induction of anaesthesia was performed using propofol with neuromuscular blockade induced with a 1mg/kg dose of rocuronium. Bag-mask ventilation proved difficult in this case. The soft tissue in the right side of the neck and mandible was very dense, and the anaesthetist found it hard to perform a jaw thrust. A two-person technique had to be used, aided by a Guedel oropharyngeal airway.

Direct laryngoscopy was performed with a size 4 Macintosh blade. A swollen and erythematous epiglottis was seen on laryngoscopy, along with copious pus within the oropharynx surrounding the epiglottis. Despite best efforts, the vocal cords or arytenoid cartilages could not be visualised. Subsequently, the anaesthetist passed a gum elastic bougie blindly under the epiglottis. He felt clicks suggesting the bougie was in the correct position. The trachea was then successfully intubated with a size 8mm ID reinforced tracheal tube. Correct placement of the tube was confirmed using capnography. The surgical drainage of the abscess was uneventful.

What is the plan for extubation in this case?

This patient had a difficult airway from the beginning. Reintubation is extremely challenging, and is likely to be impossible. In addition, there is the risk of airway obstruction due to airway oedema or worsening pathology. Therefore, it was decided to postpone extubation until the airway pathology improved. The patient was transferred to the intensive care unit (ICU), where he remained sedated and ventilated for 48 hours. Awake extubation was then performed, which was uneventful.

How would you manage this case differently?

- A thorough pre-assessment (history and examination) can identify features of difficult bag-mask ventilation alongside difficult intubation. Communicating a clear airway management strategy would limit risks to the patient.
- A flexible nasendoscopy should be performed to assess the airway before induction of anaesthesia.
- The airway management strategy should include an awake technique, such as awake tracheal intubation with a flexible fibrescope or hyperangulated blade videolaryngoscope.

3

- High-flow nasal oxygen should be administered as early as possible.
- In a situation in which the awake technique is not possible, with high-risk general anaesthesia, video-assisted fibreoptic intubation (VAFI) could be the first choice. In a situation with limited mouth opening, video-assisted nasal fibreoptic intubation would have been a better choice.
- An experienced surgeon should be scrubbed and ready to perform front-of-neck access.
- Blind insertion of a bougie is discouraged as it can cause further airway trauma. Therefore, in this case, with a grade 4 view on direct laryngoscopy, alternative techniques of laryngoscopy using a hyperangulated videolaryngoscope or VAFI should be considered.
- A clear extubation plan should be documented with consideration of additional post-procedure airway oedema from airway manipulation.

Difficult mask ventilation

Documenting the difficulty in bag-mask ventilation (Table 1.1) may aid anaesthetists in planning airway management if the patient returns to the theatre for any additional procedure in the future. Box 1.1 shows the management options for patients with difficult bag-mask ventilation.

Table 1.1. Han scale of face mask ventilation.	
Degree of difficulty	**Description**
Grade 1	Single-handed mask ventilation achieved
Grade 2	Difficult to ventilate, use of nasopharyngeal/ oropharyngeal airway required
Grade 3	Difficult mask ventilation, requiring jaw thrust, airway manoeuvres and two-handed technique
Grade 4	Unable to bag-mask ventilate

Box 1.1. Management techniques for difficult bag-mask ventilation.

1. Optimising patient positioning and reattempting airway opening manoeuvres.
2. Ensuring adequate depth of anaesthesia and considering administering muscle relaxation.
3. Use of airway adjuncts: either nasopharyngeal/oropharyngeal airway.
4. Use of continuous positive airway pressure (CPAP) to aid ventilation.
5. Use of a two-person technique.
6. Call for further help and ensure a difficult airway trolley is available.
7. Consider intubation or the use of a supraglottic airway device.
8. If a 'cannot intubate and cannot oxygenate' situation arises, consider emergency front-of-neck access.

Principles of airway management

The principles of airway management include:

- Airway assessment and anticipation of difficulty.
- Formulation of an airway management strategy.
- Performance of the procedure.
- Extubation and follow-up.
- Maintaining records and communication.

Airway assessment

Airway assessment includes a history, clinical examination and special investigations. The first consideration is whether a seal can be obtained with the face mask. A history of snoring, obstructive sleep apnoea (OSA), presence of a full beard, obesity (Box 1.2), age over 55 years, poor Mallampati grade, a thyromental distance less than 6.5cm, and poor mandibular protrusion are all associated with difficult face mask ventilation.

> **Box 1.2. Patient factors leading to difficult bag-mask ventilation.**
>
> - B — Bearded.
> - O — Obese.
> - N — No teeth.
> - E — Elderly.
> - S — Sleep apnoea.

Poor dentition, loose teeth and protruding upper teeth can make laryngoscopy difficult. A systematic review of the Cochrane database on airway assessment tests in 2018 has shown that the upper lip bite test has the highest sensitivity for predicting difficult laryngoscopy. The inability to protrude the lower teeth beyond the top teeth suggests difficult laryngoscopy.

Adequate mouth opening is important for two reasons. Firstly, to allow the passage of a laryngoscope blade in order to get a view of the glottis. Secondly, if there is a failed intubation, a supraglottic airway device (SAD) may need to be inserted to facilitate oxygenation, which may be hindered by impaired mouth opening. The normal lower limit of mouth opening (measured as inter-incisor distance) for young adults is 3.7cm (approximately three finger breadths).

With the Mallampati test, the patient is asked to open their mouth maximally and protrude their tongue without phonation while the examiner sits opposite them at the same level. The oropharynx is inspected and, depending on what is seen, there are four classes:

- Class 1: posterior pharyngeal wall visible, including the posterior pillars and the whole of the uvula, including the tip.
- Class 2: posterior pharyngeal wall visible, including the posterior pillars and part of the uvula.
- Class 3: posterior pharyngeal wall not visible and soft palate visible.
- Class 4: soft palate not visible and hard palate visible.

The combination of Mallampati Class 3 or 4, an inter-incisor distance of less than 3.7cm and a thyromental distance of less than 6.5cm, has been shown to have an 85% sensitivity and 95% specificity for difficult tracheal intubation. In addition, limited neck movements and limited neck extension can contribute to difficult laryngoscopy and difficult intubation. No tests are perfect by themselves, but combining all the information above from the history and examination will identify the groups of patients who will present a challenge in their airway management.

Special investigations

In selected patients, cervical spine X-rays (to assess craniocervical mobility), or CT and MRI scans (to assess airway patency and pathology), and flexible nasendoscopy are useful in airway assessment and planning.

Formulation of an airway management strategy

Based on airway assessment, a series of plans should be formulated and implemented as planned during airway management. A well-thought-out and appropriately executed plan is likely to result in a safe outcome. Planning for airway management involves choosing the best suited equipment, choosing a technique (awake or asleep), an experienced operator, and communicating decisions to the surgical and theatre team. The primary plan is the plan that has the highest success of securing an airway on the first attempt and is the safest approach for the patient. At least one back-up plan should be worked out in advance. This should also be appropriately communicated with the team. These plans should be explained to the patient in advance. Most important is the decision-making process whereby the failure of Plan A is recognised, and Plan B is executed. Persistent attempts at the initial technique and failure to move on to Plan B may cause increasing difficulty and more harm to the patient.

Performance of the procedure

Optimum technique, performed by an experienced operator, is very important for success in airway management.

In an anticipated difficult airway without upper airway obstruction, there are various options available. In some elective cases presenting for surgery, surgery can be safely performed under regional anaesthesia. However, a back-up airway management plan must be worked out in advance. If the patient needs general anaesthesia, then the awake technique is the safest option. This can be used using awake fibreoptic intubation or awake videolaryngoscopy. Some patients may require awake tracheostomy or front-of-neck access. An awake technique may not be possible in patients with an altered level of consciousness, patients who are uncooperative, if the patient is a child or the patient has severe learning disabilities.

In an anticipated difficult airway with upper airway obstruction, it is important to recognise the presence of airway obstruction. The site, extent and possible nature or cause should be ascertained. The patient may have pre-existing progressive airway pathology and may present with a critical airway. Ventilation may become ineffective, and patients may develop clinical signs secondary to hypoxia and hypercapnia. The presence of stridor indicates that the airway diameter is reduced by 50%. Generally, an inspiratory stridor indicates airway obstruction above the level of the vocal cords, and an expiratory stridor indicates obstruction below the level of the vocal cords. Difficulty in swallowing with drooling saliva suggests pharyngeal pathology. Dyspnoea and hoarseness of voice suggest pathology at the glottic level.

Management includes rapid airway assessment and administration of high-flow nasal oxygen. The patient should be positioned in a sitting position. Administration of nebulised adrenaline and steroids may help to reduce airway oedema in the presence of acute inflammation. A flexible nasendoscopy helps to evaluate the site and extent of glottic and supraglottic lesions. This should be performed by an experienced ENT surgeon or anaesthetist with experience in managing difficult airways.

A decision should be made whether to secure an airway awake or sleep. In either case, an experienced ENT surgeon should be gowned and ready to perform a surgical airway.

In a subglottic airway obstruction, if the upper airway is normal, most patients can be intubated following induction of general anaesthesia using a videolaryngoscope. If the level of obstruction and diameter of the tracheal lumen is known, then an appropriately sized tracheal tube can be selected.

Awake flexible fibreoptic endoscopy helps in the dynamic evaluation of airway diameter, site of obstruction and tube selection. In some patients who have a significantly narrowed tracheal lumen, extracorporeal oxygenation may be the only option.

Unanticipated difficult tracheal intubation

This is a situation in which airway management was assessed and planned easily. However, following the induction of anaesthesia, the primary plan of intubation may fail. At this stage, a safe technique to oxygenate the patient is of paramount importance. Failure to oxygenate can result in hypoxic brain damage and death. The Difficult Airway Society guidelines for the management of an unanticipated difficult tracheal intubation (Figure 1.1) are based on a series of escalating management plans: if Plan A does not work, back-up plans B, C or D must be executed.

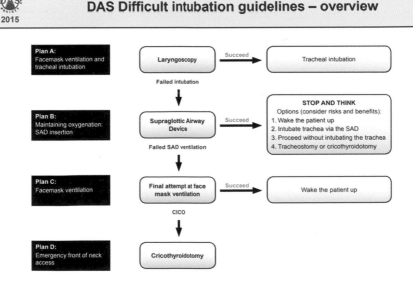

Figure 1.1. Difficult Airway Society difficult intubation guidelines: an overview. *Reproduced with permission from the Difficult Airway Society, © 2015.*

Plan A is tracheal intubation. When it fails, Plan B should be executed. Plan B involves maintaining oxygenation using a SAD. Once the SAD is inserted successfully, the decision should be made as to whether to wake the patient or to intubate the trachea through the supraglottic airway. An experienced anaesthetist can perform tracheal intubation through the supraglottic airway. In some situations, the decision to continue a life-saving surgery using a supraglottic airway may be essential. In other rare scenarios, a tracheostomy may be required at this stage.

Plan C involves an optimum attempt at oxygenation using a face mask and adjuncts.

Plan D involves rescue techniques for a 'cannot intubate, cannot oxygenate' situation. When the above methods are unsuccessful, when the patient cannot be successfully oxygenated using a face mask or supraglottic airway, the patient requires rapid surgical access to the trachea for adequate ventilation and oxygenation. Immediate recognition of this situation, a call for help, and preparation for a surgical/transtracheal airway, most commonly a cricothyroidotomy, is essential for a successful outcome.

Extubation and follow-up

Extubation can be more hazardous than intubation; therefore, it should be carefully planned. The extubation technique, the timing of extubation and a plan for reintubation if the need arises should be clearly documented. In situations in which intubation has been difficult, a follow-up interview with the patient is essential. Details of the difficulty experienced in airway management and a safe plan for future airway management must be communicated to the patient. This should be documented in their medical records. For the benefit of future airway management, there should be a mechanism whereby the information is available for the future anaesthetist. In the United Kingdom, the patient can be registered on the Difficult Airway Society database (https://das.uk.com/dad), whereby the patient can receive an alert card (Figure 1.2). The other methods include writing a letter to the patient, with a copy to their general practitioner, in addition to ensuring that the details are available in the local hospital database.

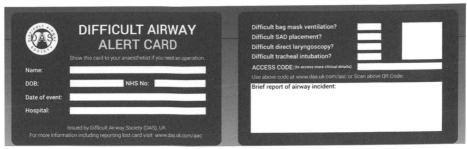

Figure 1.2. Difficult Airway Society (DAS) alert card. *Reproduced with permission from the Difficult Airway Society, © Difficult Airway Society.*

Key points

- A difficult airway has been defined by the American Society of Anesthesiologists Task Force as 'unanticipated difficulty or failure... including but not limited to one or more of the following: face mask ventilation, laryngoscopy, ventilation via a SAD, tracheal intubation, extubation or invasive airway'. A thorough airway assessment will highlight potential difficulties.
- It is important to have an airway management strategy, and this should include human factor aspects such as the most experienced operator taking the leadership role, considering various options and choosing the one best suited to the situation, and delegating the tasks to the team members.
- Delayed extubation should be considered in a patient with a known difficult airway secondary to patient factors and pathology.

References

1. Apfelbaum JL, Hagberg CA, Connis RT, *et al.* American Society of Anesthesiologists Practice Guidelines for Management of the Difficult Airway. *Anesthesiology* 2022; 136(1): 31-81.

2.   Han R, Tremper KK, Kheterpal S, O'Reilly M. Grading scale for mask ventilation. *Anesthesiology* 2004; 101(1): 267.

3.   Khan MF, Shamim F, Slote MU, *et al.* Combined use of a videolaryngoscope and a flexible bronchoscope for awake tracheal intubation when front-of-neck airway is not an option. *Anaesth Rep* 2021; 9(1): 12-5.

4.   Langeron O, Masso E, Huraux C, *et al.* Prediction of difficult mask ventilation. *Anesthesiology* 2000; 92(5): 1229-36.

5.   Nedrud SM, Baasch DG, Cabral JD, *et al.* Combined video laryngoscope and fiberoptic nasal intubation. *Cureus* 2021; 13(11): e19482.

6.   Roth D, Pace NL, Lee A, *et al.* Airway physical examination tests for detection of difficult airway management in apparently normal adult patients. *Cochrane Database Syst Rev* 2018; 5(5): CD008874.

Case scenario 2

Introduction

A 51-year-old male patient was transferred from a district general hospital to the emergency department in a tertiary teaching hospital with a history of profuse bleeding from the mouth.

Handover from the transferring team revealed that the patient had been transfused 4 units of blood and had been administered 1g of tranexamic acid. Of note, on arrival, there were a further 2 units of blood in progress, giving a total of 6 units transfused.

Past medical history

A review of the clinical records revealed that he had been diagnosed with carcinoma of the right tonsil 4 months before admission. Radical radiotherapy treatment was commenced, with his last dose being administered 3 days before admission.

Clinical examination

There was evidence of profuse bleeding within the oropharynx, with the patient lying in the left lateral position with vomit bowls containing blood clots. High-flow oxygen was administered at 15L/minute; however, oxygen was frequently removed to allow further vomiting.

He appeared pale and clammy and remained responsive to a voice. His pulse rate was 110 bpm. Systolic blood pressure measurements were persistently 70–80mmHg, despite ongoing fluid resuscitation. Mouth opening and neck movements appeared normal. Further airway assessments could not be performed due to airway soiling.

Investigations

His arterial blood gas results on admission were as shown below (on 15L/minute of oxygen)(Box 2.1).

Box 2.1. Arterial blood gas results on admission.		
	Results	**Normal**
pH	7.19	7.35–7.45
PaO_2	35.9kPa	11.9–13.3kPa
$PaCO_2$	4.16kPa	4.7–6.0kPa
Bicarbonate	20.8mmol/L	22–26mmol/L
Base excess	−4.8	−2 to +2
Lactate	6mmol/L	<2mmol/L
SaO_2	99%	94–99%
Hb	106g/L	130–160g/L

He was deemed too haemodynamically unstable to undergo a CT angiogram at this time.

The initial management of this patient

- The major haemorrhage protocol was initiated, and fluid was administered via a level 1 infuser (Belmont® Rapid Infuser). Pack 1 (containing 4 units of packed red cells and 4 units of fresh frozen plasma) and Pack 2 (containing 4 units of packed red cells, 4 units of fresh frozen plasma and 2 units of platelets) were administered. A further 1g of tranexamic acid was administered.
- The anaesthetic and the maxillofacial consultant were contacted and asked to urgently attend the theatre.

- Once it was known they were present on site, the decision was made to transfer the patient to a theatre for airway protection and haemorrhage control. The massive blood transfusion was in progress throughout the transfer.

What potential aetiologies could cause bleeding in the airway?

Box 2.2 gives a differential diagnosis for the potential aetiologies that may cause bleeding in the upper airway.

Box 2.2. Causes of upper airway bleeding.

- Spontaneous from the nasal mucosa.
- Trauma to the oropharynx, airway.
- Malignancy: nasal, oropharyngeal and laryngeal tumours.
- Vascular malformations.
- Bleeding disorder and thrombolysis.
- Surgical: following nasal and oropharyngeal surgery.
- Iatrogenic: following instrumentation of the airway, insertion of a nasogastric tube and nasal intubation.

How could blood within the upper airway make your management more difficult?

- There is a high risk of failure of airway management; the most experienced staff members are required to increase the chance of first-pass intubation.
- Increased stress levels in staff; therefore, there may be potentially less situational awareness.
- The choice of equipment may vary and blood may render videolaryngoscopes less useful. It would also be difficult to visualise structures using a fibreoptic scope.

- A definitive airway is required to avoid a risk of aspiration, which renders supraglottic devices not suitable.
- Pre-oxygenation may be more difficult. The use of high-flow nasal oxygenation would be relatively contraindicated as it may worsen bleeding by disrupting the blood clots.
- Often a time-critical intervention is needed to gain haemostasis and prevent further haemodynamic instability or allow fluid resuscitation to be more effective. This will often require multiple personnel available to help manage the patient.
- The use of suction devices may limit the working space within the oral cavity.
- Unable to lie the patient flat while awake; patients may prefer a sitting position to avoid the feeling of suffocation.
- 'Waking the patient' following failed airway intervention may not be an option.
- The patient may rebleed on extubation, so a clear plan needs to be made before extubation.

How this case was managed

Following discussions between the anaesthetic consultant and maxillofacial consultant, it was decided to attempt oral tracheal intubation under general anaesthesia with a team scrubbed for emergency tracheostomy insertion.

For preparation, the difficult airway trolley was brought into the theatre and a single-use fibrescope (Ambu® aScope™) was available if required. Because of the amount of airway soiling, an airway plan was formed and communicated:

- Plan A was a rapid sequence induction with two suction catheters and direct laryngoscopy (Macintosh 4 blade).
- Plan B was a reattempt with continuous suctioning with a videolaryngoscope.
- Plan C was to hand over to a surgeon for front-of-neck access with a surgical tracheostomy.

General anaesthesia was induced with an intravenous induction using ketamine (1mg/kg) and rocuronium (1mg/kg). The first attempt at laryngoscopy using direct laryngoscopy with a Macintosh 4 blade revealed a grade III view of the glottis, with pooling of fresh blood in the oropharynx. A bougie was inserted and a tracheal tube was 'railroaded' over the bougie; however, there was no capnography trace visible. Therefore, the tube was removed. As the tube was being withdrawn, a capnography waveform was seen on the monitor. Unfortunately, at this time, the tube was completely out of the trachea.

A second attempt at laryngoscopy was performed with a McGrath™ videolaryngoscope using a size 4 Mac blade with continuous suctioning. A grade IV view was seen on this occasion; therefore, a decision was made to proceed with a surgical tracheostomy. Despite the surgeon visually confirming the tracheostomy tube was in the trachea, there was no capnography trace visible. After a long delay, the capnography trace appeared. Of note, throughout all attempts, the patient's oxygen saturation remained at 100%, and the team was able to bag-mask ventilate as a rescue strategy.

Intra-operative findings

Examination under anaesthesia revealed that the tumour had invaded the lateral pharynx, with clots overlying the tonsillar bed and a generalised ooze. A bleeding vessel was evident on the medial aspect of the parapharyngeal space.

Postoperative management

A bronchoscopy was performed in the theatre. Frank clots were removed from the patient's bronchial tree. He was subsequently transferred to the intensive care unit (ICU) as a level 3 critical-care support for ongoing stabilisation. Once stabilised, an MRI scan was performed to assess the

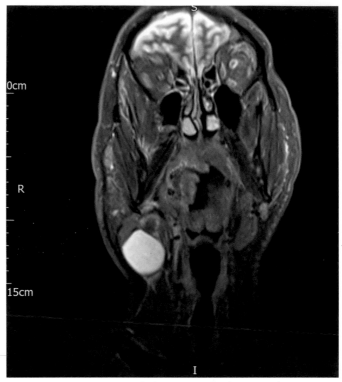

Figure 2.1. MRI scan of the coronal plane. Malignancy is shown *in situ* with evidence of invasion of local structures and causing a deformity of the upper airway.

extent of underlying airway pathology (Figures 2.1 and 2.2). A CT scan confirmed a large ulcerated invasive right tonsillar tumour invading the tongue base, the floor of the mouth, the lateral pharyngeal wall and extrinsic tongue muscles. On review of his previous records, he had a CT scan 3 months earlier, which confirmed a T4aN2b right oropharyngeal malignancy.

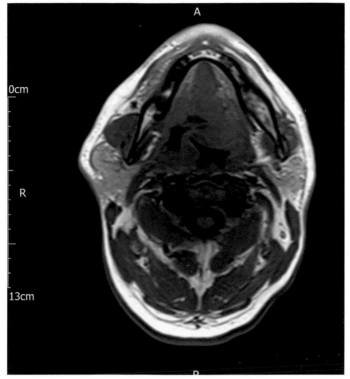

Figure 2.2. MRI scan in the transverse plane.

Why was there no capnography trace initially on tracheal intubation?

On intubation, despite feeling tracheal rings with the bougie, no capnography trace was seen for a prolonged period. Because of the Royal College of Anaesthetists' campaign 'no trace, wrong place', a decision was therefore made to remove the tracheal tube. Subsequently, following the insertion of the tracheostomy tube, there was a significant delay in the appearance of a capnography trace. In this case, the most likely reason for the absence of a capnography trace was a large blood clot contributing to a ball valve mechanism. During the inspiratory phase of positive pressure ventilation, the clot is dislodged away from the tip of the tracheal tube and, during the expiratory phase, it blocks the tip of the tracheal tube. This emphasises the relevance of considering a differential diagnosis for the absence of a capnography trace. Although incorrect tracheal tube placement is the most likely cause, other causes include breathing system disconnection; complete airway obstruction due to blood clots in the tube or trachea should be ruled out.

How would you manage this case differently?

- The Suction-Assisted Laryngoscopy and Decontamination (SALAD) technique could be utilised to optimise the view at laryngoscopy to aid first-pass successful intubation.
- Consideration of awake tracheostomy as plan A to avoid further trauma to the oropharyngeal lesion.
- Awareness of the causes of delayed capnography traces; consideration of the use of adjuncts to confirm tracheal tube placement such as bronchoscopy. Ensure that a bronchoscope is immediately available.

Management strategy for a patient with a bleeding airway

- Compress the bleeding site if possible.
- Place the patient in a head up position.
- Gentle suction and high-flow oxygen via a face mask.
- Fluid resuscitation with transfusion of blood products.
- Assess the airway, identify the cricothyroid membrane and ensure that an experienced ENT surgeon is ready and that equipment for a tracheostomy or front-of-neck access is immediately available.
- If airway management is predicted to be easy, perform a rapid sequence induction of general anaesthesia and intubation. If this fails, the next option should be front-of-neck access (either cricothyroidotomy or tracheostomy).
- If airway management is predicted to be difficult, an awake technique such as awake front-of-neck access/tracheostomy should

be considered. Awake fibreoptic and awake videolaryngoscopy can be challenging in the presence of active bleeding.

Key points

- Optimisation of the view at laryngoscopy will reduce the risk of inadvertent oesophageal intubation. The presence of blood in the airway can cause difficulty in the visualisation of anatomical structures.
- Awareness of human factor-related issues that contribute to critical incidents and actively delegating tasks reduces the cognitive load on the person intubating and improves patient management. Effective multidisciplinary planning and appropriate mobilisation of resources are essential.
- There is a significant risk of aspiration of swallowed blood from the stomach.
- Hypovolaemia from blood loss can compound haemodynamic stability. The patient may be extremely agitated from both hypovolaemia and hypoxia.
- Waking the patient from the failed airway management is not an option in this scenario.

References

1. DuCanto J, Serrano KD, Thompson RJ. Novel airway training tool that simulates vomiting: suction-assisted laryngoscopy assisted decontamination (SALAD) system. *West J Emerg Med* 2017; 18(1): 117-20.

2. Kristensen MS, McGuire B. Managing and securing the bleeding upper airway: a narrative review. *Can J Anaesth* 2020; 67(1): 128-40.

3. Royal College of Anaesthetists. Capnography: no trace = wrong place; 2018. Available from: https://www.rcoa.ac.uk/safety-standards-quality/guidance-resources/capnography-no-trace-wrong-place.

Case scenario 3

Introduction

A 45-year-old woman was referred urgently to the emergency department by her general practitioner with a suspicion of acute epiglottitis. She was brought to the hospital by ambulance, accompanied by two relatives. The main presenting complaints were a sore throat, difficulties in breathing and an inability to swallow. The symptoms gradually increased in severity over a period of hours.

Past medical history

- Multinodular goitre with associated hyperthyroidism, being managed by endocrinology.
- Anxiety.

Clinical examination

From a distance, she was noted to have saliva drooling from her mouth but was conscious and cooperative. She was speaking in broken sentences with a weak voice. She was noted to be pink and warm to the touch.

Her observations were as follows:

- Apyrexial.
- Respiratory rate was 25 breaths/minute.
- Oxygen saturation was 97% in room air.
- Heart rate was 100 beats/minute.
- Blood pressure was 135/80mmHg.

A moderate sized goitre was palpable on examination.

Investigations

A review of previous medical records showed that the recent thyroid stimulating hormone (TSH) was low and the levels of tri-iodothyronine (T3) and tetra-iodothyronine (T4) were moderately elevated. The patient, however, did not attend her last endocrinology appointment.

How this case was managed

Treatment was commenced immediately with intravenous antibiotics and steroids. Nebulised adrenaline was administered with no improvement in the patient's condition. Half an hour after the admission to the hospital, the patient lost the ability to phonate and several minutes later, she developed stridor.

The anaesthetist and an ENT surgeon were requested to attend. At this point, an airway assessment revealed:

- Normal mouth opening.
- Mallampati score of 2.
- Full dentition.
- Normal range of neck movements.

What method of securing the airway was chosen in this case?

The patient was transferred to the anaesthetic room of the emergency theatre with the intention of performing a flexible nasendoscopy and assess the airway pathology.

A fibreoptic bronchoscope was inserted into the patient's nostril, but she could not tolerate the procedure and moved violently.

What was the next step?

To help with the discomfort, the nasal mucosa was anaesthetised with a mixture of 5% lidocaine and 0.5% phenylephrine. This produced no improvement.

Therefore, sedation with intravenous alfentanil and midazolam was commenced in small incremental doses.

Immediately, there was a marked improvement in the intensity of stridor. Soon afterwards, the stridor disappeared altogether, as did all the other signs of respiratory distress. The naso-endoscopic view of the pharynx and larynx was normal, with no signs of inflammation or other pathology. It was felt the stridor was a presentation of Munchausen syndrome. The potential differential diagnosis for stridor is shown in Table 3.1.

Table 3.1. Differential diagnosis of stridor.

Infection: epiglottitis/retropharyngeal abscess	Malignancy: oral/laryngeal
Foreign body in the airway	Laryngeal oedema from anaphylaxis and inhalational injury
Bilateral vocal cord palsy	External compression from a neck haematoma, goitre, malignant lymph nodes
Retropharyngeal haematoma: post-tracheostomy stenosis	
	Iatrogenic: post-intubation stenosis
Inflammatory: cricoarytenoid rheumatoid arthritis	Munchausen syndrome

How would you manage this case differently?

- A thorough review of the clinical records revealed previous medical alerts and multiple previous hospital admissions suggestive of Munchausen syndrome. The sudden deterioration following nebulised adrenaline may be a warning sign that this may not be a pathological process.
- Consider a carefully titrated dose of shorter-acting sedative agents such as propofol or remifentanil along with high-flow nasal oxygenation and full monitoring to allow flexible nasendoscopy.
- Use of temporising measures such as:
  - high-flow nasal cannulae to pre-oxygenate;
  - the use of Heliox to improve flow across the upper airway.
- Consider ongoing treatment for Munchausen syndrome.

Key points

- Respiratory distress has been described as a potential presentation of Munchausen syndrome. Some of these cases have been subsequently intubated for airway protection.
- Reassess the diagnosis if there is no response to conventional treatment and rule out any acute airway pathology.
- Further treatment will be determined by whether the patient accepts the diagnosis. They may benefit from psychiatric input or cognitive behavioural therapy. If they do not accept, the best course of action is to minimise medicalising the patient.

References

1. Lynch J, Crawley SM. Management of airway obstruction. *BJA Educ* 2018; 18(2): 46-51.
2. NHS UK. Overview of Munchausen's syndrome. Available from: https://www.nhs.uk/mental-health/conditions/munchausens-syndrome/overview/.
3. Rafter AT, Lim E, Östör AJK, Eds. *Churchill's Pocketbook of Differential Diagnosis*, 4th ed. Elsevier/Churchill Livingstone; 2014.

Case scenario 4

Introduction

A 39-year-old woman was admitted to the hospital for an elective lumbar microdiscectomy. She had a history of severe radicular lower back pain and progressive sensory deficit in both legs.

Past medical history

- Class 3 obesity with a body mass index (BMI) of 45kg/m^2.
- She had no other coexisting diseases.

Clinical examination

An airway assessment was performed that showed:

- A Mallampati score of 3.
- The mobility of the neck was good.
- Jaw protrusion of Class A and was able to protrude the lower teeth beyond the top teeth.

When asked about previous surgeries, the patient said that she had undergone an umbilical hernia repair 4 years before. She was not informed about any problems with the anaesthetic.

Investigations

A review of the previous anaesthetic chart revealed a Cormack and Lehane grade 3 view of the larynx with direct laryngoscopy. No other details on the intubation were provided.

How this case was managed

A ramped-up position was used using an Oxford HELP® pillow. It was ensured that the external auditory meatus was aligned with the suprasternal notch in the horizontal plane, as demonstrated in Figure 4.1. Routine intravenous induction of anaesthesia was performed, followed by an intubating dose of atracurium. Face mask ventilation was easy.

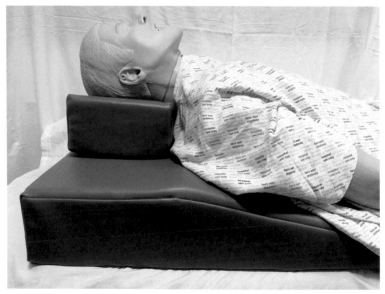

Figure 4.1. Ramped position achieved using an Oxford HELP® pillow.

An asleep fibreoptic-guided intubation was attempted via the oral route by an anaesthetic registrar. They found the procedure difficult, and oxygen saturation started to drop before they could visualise the vocal cords. Therefore, an oropharyngeal airway was inserted, and the face mask ventilation was recommenced. A second attempt at fibreoptic intubation was made by a consultant anaesthetist, who also failed to visualise the vocal cords before the oxygen saturation started dropping.

What was the next step?

Face mask ventilation was restarted, general anaesthesia was maintained and help was requested. A consultant with an airway interest attended promptly and decided to attempt intubation using a McGrath™ videolaryngoscope with a MAC 4 blade. In total, 50% of the glottis could be visualised on the screen. When taking a direct look, only the tip of the epiglottis was visible. A bougie was successfully passed into the trachea under videolaryngoscopic view and a reinforced tracheal tube 'railroaded' over the bougie. Correct placement of the tracheal tube was confirmed using capnography.

How would you manage this case differently?

- To facilitate oxygenation, supplemental oxygen therapy could have been used as pre-oxygenation, for example, high-flow nasal oxygen.
- As this was an elective procedure, oxygenation could have been achieved with a supraglottic airway device and the patient could have been woken up and rescheduled to have awake tracheal intubation at a later stage on the same day or another day.
- The management of this case shows the difficult airway algorithm (Figure 1.1) was followed as expected. This gives an example of how our thinking may be influenced by whether we recognise if a situation is progressing well or badly. This may influence how

quickly we reach a decision. Situational awareness and a decision-making ability are essential non-technical skills in an emergency.

Most medics work through difficult clinical conundrums using pattern recognition. This can either lead to quick decision making through intuitive thinking if the pattern is recognised or slower analytical thinking if the pattern is not recognised. This can, in turn, lead to quicker or slower overall decision making.

Multiple factors can change whether we think intuitively or analytically, such as repetition, thinking things through logically (executive override) or thinking irrationally (irrational override). Before making a decision, we generally confirm our choice by calibrating our thoughts to the scenario we are faced with.

Using protocols and by practising emergency scenarios, we hope to instil intuitive thinking into our general practice rather than analytical thinking, allowing us to have the best patient outcome with the shortest delay.

Key points

- To some, the decision making in this case may seem to err on the side of caution. It is easy to feel tempted to make another attempt at fibreoptic intubation or try direct laryngoscopy. The anaesthetist demonstrated good situational awareness and avoided making multiple repeated attempts at intubation. They requested help on time. A change of equipment and an operator resulted in successful tracheal intubation.
- Within the UK, the high-profile case of Elaine Bromiley highlighted how to avoid adverse events. We need to be aware of human factors that can affect our daily work.

References

1. Bromiley M. Have you ever made a mistake? *R Coll Anaesth Bull* 2008; 48: 2442-5.

2. Gibbins M, Kelly FE, Cook TM. Airway management equipment and practice: time to optimise institutional, team, and personal preparedness. *Br J Anaesth* 2020; 125(3): 221-4.

3. Stiegler MP, Tung A. Cognitive processes in anesthesiology decision making. *Anesthesiology* 2014; 120(1): 204-17.

Case scenario 5

Introduction

A 69-year-old female patient presented on an elective operating list for radiofrequency ablation of a liver lesion. In addition to the liver lesion, she was noted not to have any other medical conditions.

Past history

She had no other past medical history to note.

Clinical examination

During the pre-operative visit, an airway assessment was performed:

- She had limited neck extension.
- Mallampati score of 2.
- She was relatively short, with a height of 152cm, and had a raised BMI of 32kg/m^2.

Investigations

The results of pre-operative haematology and biochemistry tests were within the normal range.

How this case was managed

The anaesthetist decided to induce general anaesthesia and perform tracheal intubation using direct laryngoscopy as Plan A. Plan B was to use a channelled videolaryngoscope. Following pre-oxygenation, general anaesthesia was induced intravenously with fentanyl and propofol and followed by a standard dose of non-depolarising muscle relaxant. Direct laryngoscopy was performed with a Macintosh blade. The anaesthetist encountered a grade 4 Cormack and Lehane view of the glottis. External

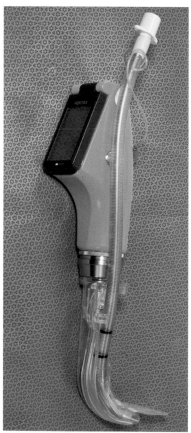

Figure 5.1. Pentax Airway Scope (AWS®) (Pentax Corporation, Tokyo, Japan) channelled videolaryngoscope.

laryngeal manipulation using backward, upward, rightward pressure (BURP) did not improve the view.

The anaesthetist resumed face mask ventilation, and a channelled videolaryngoscope (Pentax Airway Scope [AWS®], Pentax Corporation, Tokyo, Japan) was prepared by the assistant (Figure 5.1). The blade of the videolaryngoscope was easy to insert into the mouth, but again, neither the glottis nor the epiglottis could be visualised. Following two failed laryngoscopy attempts, a failed intubation was declared, and the anaesthetist inserted a size 4 i-gel® supraglottic airway device as per the Difficult Airway Society guidelines for managing unanticipated difficult intubation (Figure 5.2). It was easy to ventilate via a supraglottic airway device; additional help was summoned.

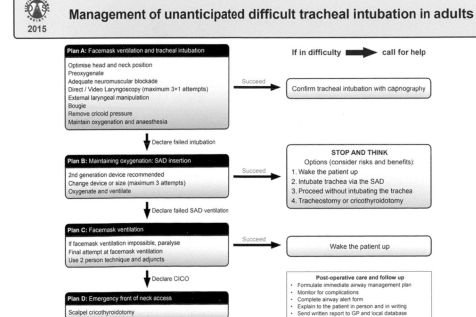

Figure 5.2. Management of unanticipated difficult tracheal intubation in adults. *Reproduced with permission from the Difficult Airway Society, © 2015.*

What was the next step?

At this stage, the patient was well oxygenated using a supraglottic airway device. The surgical procedure required general anaesthesia with tracheal intubation. A second anaesthetist with expertise in difficult airway management arrived promptly. He requested the assistant to collect a fibreoptic bronchoscope and a second, non-channelled videolaryngoscope with a hyperangulated blade (C-MAC® D-Blade, Karl Storz, Tuttlingen, Germany). First, the anaesthetist was delegated the task of monitoring the patient and maintaining anaesthesia with intravenous boluses of propofol. The second anaesthetist then performed fibreoptic endoscopy through the supraglottic airway device and obtained a good view of the vocal cords. A decision was then made to perform a two-stage fibreoptic-guided intubation using an Aintree intubation catheter (AIC), as shown in Figure 5.3. The stages of the two-stage procedure were as follows:

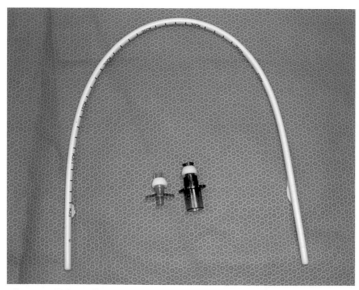

Figure 5.3. Aintree intubating catheter with Rapi-Fit® connectors.

- A laryngeal mask airway (LMA) was inserted to ensure adequate ventilation was possible.

- The AIC was loaded onto the fibreoptic bronchoscope that was passed through the i-gel®. The AIC was placed in the trachea above the carina.

- The fibrescope and i-gel® were removed, leaving the AIC in the trachea. At this point a Rapi-Fit® connector could be attached, allowing the patient to be ventilated.

- In this case, laryngoscopy using a C-MAC® videolaryngoscope with a hyperangulated blade (D-Blade) was then performed to confirm that the AIC had not been displaced during the removal of the i-gel® (Figure 5.4). This gave a 75% view of the glottic opening.

- A size 7.5mm tracheal tube was 'railroaded' over the AIC and the capnography trace confirmed its placement in the trachea. A 90° rotation of the tracheal tube may be required to avoid impingement at the vocal cords.

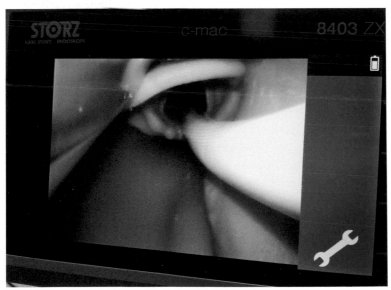

Figure 5.4. View on a videolaryngoscope of the AIC passing through the vocal cords into the trachea.

Postoperative management

The patient was visited by the second anaesthetist, who assessed the airway in more detail. A repeat airway assessment confirmed that a difficult airway could have been anticipated for this patient:

- An inter-incisor gap of 4cm.
- The thyromental distance was normal at 7.5cm.
- Neck circumference was noted at 40cm.
- Limited ability to protrude the jaw, with Class B mandibular protrusion (the lower incisor could just meet the upper incisors on jaw protrusion).
- Limited neck extension.
- Sternomental distance of 12cm was borderline.
- A thyroidectomy scar was visible on the patient's neck.

Further enquiry about her surgical history revealed a history of thyroidectomy 8 years ago with a history of difficult tracheal intubation. In the first instance, the operation was cancelled because of a failed tracheal intubation. The surgery was then rescheduled and, on the second occasion, awake fibreoptic intubation was likely to have been performed. Unfortunately, the anaesthetic chart was not available in the patient's medical records.

Following a re-examination of the patient, multiple factors were identified that could suggest this patient would have difficult intubation. The 4th National Audit Project of the Royal College of Anaesthetists and the Difficult Airway Society has shown that poor assessment was deemed to be the commonest contributory factor to poor airway management. Although there is no definition of what comprises an 'adequate' airway assessment, it generally comprises a history of previous difficulties, gaining a history of medical conditions that may cause difficulties, such as obstructive sleep apnoea and rheumatoid arthritis, previous surgery or radiotherapy to the head and neck region alongside bedside clinical tests. Although bedside tests generally have poor predictive values, they will often dictate airway management strategies if poor neck mobility or poor mouth opening is present.

The main aim of these predictors is to allow the anaesthetist to adequately prepare for airway management. This will incorporate appropriate equipment, personnel and planning, and communicating an airway management strategy.

How would you manage this case differently?

- A thorough pre-operative assessment including a detailed history and thorough clinical examination to predict possible difficult intubation.
- A detailed explanation of a possible difficult airway and safety of the awake technique would facilitate gaining consent for awake tracheal intubation. This could be either awake fibreoptic intubation or awake videolaryngoscopy. A combination of videolaryngoscopy and fibreoptic scope can be used to improve the success of tracheal intubation.

Box 5.1. Steps to perform a one-stage tracheal intubation via a supraglottic airway device.

- Load an appropriately sized tracheal tube onto a flexible videoscope or fibreoptic scope.
- Pass the scope through the second-generation supraglottic airway device and visualise the epiglottis and vocal cords (step 1, Figure 5.5).
- Pass the scope through the vocal cords until a view of the carina is visible (step 2, Figure 5.5).
- Once the carina is visible, pass the tracheal tube over the scope until the tip is visible in a good position above the carina (step 3, Figure 5.5).
- Remove the scope from the lumen of the tracheal tube, connect the breathing circuit and confirm tube placement using capnography.
- Once confirmed, secure the tracheal tube in place. The second-generation supraglottic airway device will remain *in situ* (step 4, Figure 5.5).

- In the United Kingdom, a search of the DAS Difficult Airway Database may be useful to check for any previous entry of airway difficulty.
- A one-stage fibreoptic assisted intubation using a size 7mm tracheal tube could have been performed through an i-gel®. In this situation, a decision needs to be made whether an i-gel® needs to be removed

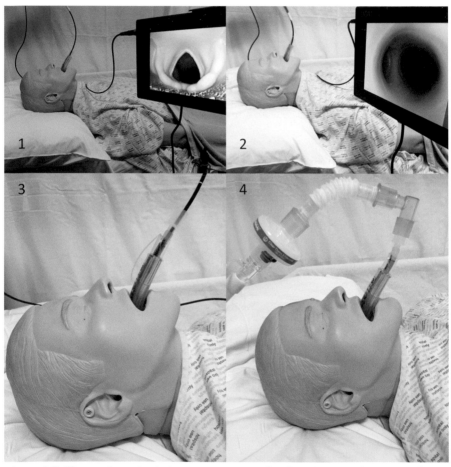

Figure 5.5. Illustrations depicting one-stage tracheal intubation via a supraglottic airway device.

or kept *in situ* for the duration of the anaesthetic. This would depend upon surgical factors such as length of operation and required patient positioning.

The steps to perform one-stage tracheal intubation via a second-generation supraglottic airway device are described in Box 5.1. These are illustrated in a stepwise manner in Figure 5.5.

Practical tips for successful fibreoptic intubation via a supraglottic airway device

- Choose an appropriately sized tracheal tube that easily passes through the ventilation tube of the supraglottic airway device. The author's choice is a single-use intubating LMA tube.
- Ensure good lubrication between the scope and fibreoptic scope and between the tube and lumen of the ventilation tube of the supraglottic airway device.
- Minimise the risk of tube impingement at the level of arytenoids by preloading the tube so that the bevel faces backwards.

If the supraglottic airway device needs to be removed for surgery or if the patient requires long-term ventilation, a two-stage technique can be used using an AIC as a conduit. This allows the supraglottic airway device to be removed and an endotracheal tube to be 'railroaded' into position.

Most currently available second-generation supraglottic airway devices have a shorter and wider ventilation tube. This characteristic facilitates the passage of tracheal tubes of size 6mm to 7.5mm ID, depending on the size and type of second-generation supraglottic airway devices (Figure 5.6).

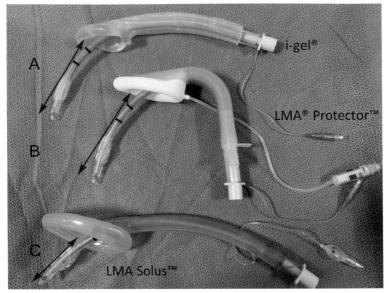

Figure 5.6. Characteristics of second-generation supraglottic airway devices facilitating tracheal intubation. Note the safe length of the tube available distal to the laryngeal aperture of the supraglottic airway device (A and B) ensures that the tracheal tube cuff is beyond the vocal cords compared with the first-generation supraglottic airway device (C).

Key points

- A thorough pre-operative history and airway assessment are important to predict potentially difficult intubation. This was emphasised in the 4th National Audit Project of the Royal College of Anaesthetists and Difficult Airway Society. A well planned airway management strategy improves the success of tracheal intubation.

- In a predicted difficult airway, awake tracheal intubation is the safest technique in securing an airway.

- The use of electronic patient records and difficult airway alerts would increase anaesthetists' awareness of previous difficult intubations.

References

1. Difficult Airway Society. DAS airway alert card and Difficult Airway Database – general information. Available from: https://das.uk.com/aac/project_information.
2. Frerk CM, Mitchell VS, McNarry AF, *et al.* Difficult Airway Society 2015 guidelines for management of unanticipated difficult intubation in adults. *Br J Anaesth* 2015; 115(6): 827-48.
3. Langeron O, Semjen F, Bourgain JL, *et al.* Comparison of the intubating laryngeal mask airway with the fiberoptic intubation in anticipated difficult airway management. *Anesthesiology* 2001; 94(6): 968-72.
4. Pearce A, Shaw J. Airway assessment and planning. In: Cook T, Woodall N, Frerk C, Eds. 4th National Audit Project of the Royal College of Anaesthetists and The Difficult Airway Society; 2011. Available from: https://www.nationalauditprojects.org.uk/downloads/Section%201.pdf.
5. Rich JM. Recognition and management of the difficult airway with special emphasis on the intubating LMA-Fastrach/whistle technique: a brief review with case reports. *Proc (Bayl Univ Med Cent)* 2005; 18(3): 220-7.
6. Sajayan A, Nair A, McNarry AF, *et al.* Analysis of a national difficult airway database. *Anaesthesia* 2022; 77(10): 1081-8.

Case scenario 6

Introduction

A 53-year-old lady presented on the elective neurosurgical list for anterior cervical discectomy and fusion to relieve symptoms of cervical spondylosis.

Past medical history

- Obesity with a BMI of 35kg/m^2.
- Type 2 diabetes mellitus.
- Hypertension.

Clinical examination

During the pre-operative visit, the anaesthetist immediately noted that she had a slightly receding chin. A more detailed airway examination showed:

- Mallampati score of 2.
- Thyromental distance of 7.5cm.
- Jaw protrusion class B; on maximal protrusion of the lower jaw, the lower incisors protruded to reach the upper incisors.
- Moderate limitation of neck extension.

Investigations

The results of pre-operative haematology and biochemistry tests were within the normal range.

How this case was managed

The anaesthetist decided to perform routine induction of anaesthesia followed by direct laryngoscopy. After standard patient monitoring was applied and intravenous access was obtained, induction of anaesthesia was performed using target-controlled infusions of remifentanil and propofol. An intubating dose of rocuronium was administered after the loss of consciousness.

On attempting face mask ventilation, the anaesthetist found that they were only able to ventilate the lungs using a two-hand technique and an oropharyngeal (Guedel) airway. This was not improved by the onset of the neuromuscular blockade. Direct laryngoscopy with a size 4 Macintosh blade showed a grade 4 Cormack-Lehane view of the glottis. A second attempt using a McCoy blade did not improve the laryngoscopic view.

The anaesthetist decided to use a supraglottic airway device to oxygenate the patient and to allow time to draft a further management plan. A size 4 i-gel® supraglottic airway was inserted without any problems. Positive pressure ventilation through the device was easy.

The surgeon was informed about the difficulties with securing the patient's airway, and a decision was made to intubate the trachea via an i-gel®.

What further equipment was asked for?

The anaesthetist chose to proceed with a fibreoptic intubation through the i-gel®.

A well lubricated, 6mm ID standard tracheal tube was loaded on the fibreoptic bronchoscope. After passing the fibrescope through the i-gel®, the vocal cords were visualised. The scope was then successfully passed through the cords into the trachea. However, this did not bring an end to the difficulties, as the anaesthetist was unable to 'railroad' the tracheal tube past the vocal cords, despite withdrawal and anticlockwise rotation of the tube. The fibreoptic bronchoscope was withdrawn, and ventilation was continued through the i-gel®.

What was the next step?

At this stage, after a discussion with the surgeon, the anaesthetist decided to abandon further attempts at securing the airway and postpone the surgery. The neuromuscular blockade was reversed with sugammadex and the patient was woken up. The surgery was rescheduled for another day when awake fibreoptic intubation was performed successfully.

How would you manage this case differently?

- Truly, this is an anticipated difficult airway. In addition, the patient may have an unstable cervical spine for which immobility of the cervical spine should be maintained during tracheal intubation. The safety of an awake technique should be explained to the patient during the pre-operative visits and consent should be obtained.

- Preparation and optimum positioning for laryngoscopy are of paramount importance for success at tracheal intubation. The use of the back-up and head-elevated laryngoscopy position (HELP) may improve the success of direct laryngoscopy. In the obese population, this may be achieved with a ramp under the patient's head and shoulders. However, in this patient, it was important to maintain the neck in a neutral position.

- The first anaesthetist should call for help early. Following three failed intubations and at a point at which oxygenation was achieved with a supraglottic airway device, the anaesthetist should stop and think. This would be in line with current DAS difficult intubation guidelines (Figure 5.2). During this stage, a mini brief should be performed involving the scrub team and surgeon. The team should explore the available options and decide on the most appropriate management option, considering patient safety as of paramount importance.

- It is important to know the correct size of the tracheal tube that can be introduced through each i-gel® (Table 6.1). However, the larger the tracheal tube, the likelihood of tube impingement at arytenoids will increase, resulting in further difficulty in intubation. As described in Case scenario 10, tube size and tube design are important for improving the success of fibreoptic-assisted tracheal intubation.

Table 6.1. Different i-gel® sizes with the largest size of tracheal tube that can be used.		
i-gel® size	Weight of patient (kg)	Size tracheal tube (mm ID)
3	30–50	6
4	50–90	7
5	>90	8

- Following the procedure, the patient should be counselled on the airway issues encountered, and written information should be added to a difficult airway database as well as provided to the patient and their general practitioner (as shown in Figure 1.2).

Key points

- A thorough pre-operative airway assessment allows us to identify features that may suggest difficult airway management.
- In an anticipated difficult airway, awake tracheal intubation is the safest technique to secure an airway.
- Limiting the number of attempts at laryngoscopy and tracheal intubation and understanding the role of human factors are of great importance during airway management.
- In a crisis, successful management and a good outcome depend on clear leadership, task delegation to team members, situational awareness and the right decisions made at the right time.
- In an elective situation, waking the patient up and rescheduling the procedure could be a safe option for the patient.

References

1. Difficult Airway Society. DAS airway alert card and Difficult Airway Database – general Information. Available from: https://das.uk.com/aac/project_information.

2. Intersurgical 2022. About the i-gel®. Available from: https://www.intersurgical.com/info/igel.

3. Sung A, Kalstein A, Radhakrishnan P, *et al.* Review article: Laryngeal mask airway: use and clinical application. *J Bronchol* 2007; 14(3): 181-8.

4. Tsan SEH, Lim SM, Abidin MFZ, *et al.* Comparison of Macintosh laryngoscopy in bed-up-head-elevated position with GlideScope laryngoscopy: a randomized, controlled, noninferiority trial. *Anesth Analg* 2020; 131(1): 210-9.

- Fracture of the temporal bone.
- Multilevel cervical spine fractures.
- There was no significant intracranial pathology.

How this case was managed

A neurosurgical consultant was consulted and felt that an operative intervention was not necessary and planned to manage the cervical spine injuries conservatively by immobilising the cervical spine with a halo ring brace.

The patient's left upper limb, however, started to show signs of vascular compromise. Prompt surgical reduction and internal fixation of the left humeral fracture were advocated, and the procedure was booked on the emergency trauma theatre list.

The surgery was anticipated to be complex and prolonged. Regional anaesthesia was deemed unsuitable because of the nature of the procedure and additional surgical procedures. Therefore, a general anaesthetic was planned with awake fibreoptic intubation to minimise the movement of the cervical spine during the airway manipulation.

Pre-operative assessment

The patient was clinically stable with no signs of respiratory distress or shock. In the past, she had undergone an uneventful general anaesthetic for a dental procedure. She was fully alert, orientated and anxious. It was clear that her anxiety levels increased greatly as the anaesthetist discussed the plan and technique for awake fibreoptic intubation.

The tracheal intubation plan

The anaesthetist encouraged the patient to express her fears. On further questioning, it was established that the visible equipment was causing her anxiety. The anaesthetist then suggested the use of an awake videolaryngoscopy, rather than an awake fibreoptic intubation and discovered that a compact videolaryngoscope was deemed more acceptable to the patient.

An awake tracheal intubation was performed with the use of a non-channelled McGrath™ X blade™ videolaryngoscope. This blade was chosen as it is a hyperangulated blade allowing a view of the cords when there are predictors for difficult intubation. The more acute angle of the blade, as shown in Figure 7.1, allows for improved glottic exposure. A target-controlled infusion of remifentanil, with target plasma concentrations of between 2 and 3ng/ml, was used to provide conscious sedation.

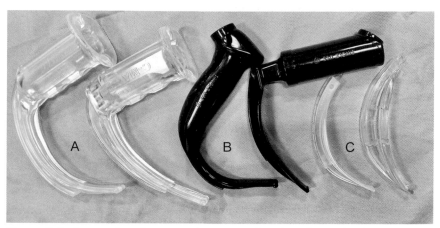

Figure 7.1. Comparison between hyperangulated and standard Macintosh style blades. A) C MAC® D-Blade and Mac blade. B) GlideScope® Spectrum™ LoPro and Mac blade. C) McGrath™ X blade™ and Mac blade.

The oropharynx was anaesthetised with an atomised local anaesthetic (4% lidocaine). The X blade™ was inserted into the oral cavity under direct vision.

Additional local anaesthetic (4% lidocaine) was administered to the epiglottis and glottis using a mucosal atomisation device (Figure 7.2). The blade was advanced further to obtain a full view of the glottis, and an additional dose of 4% lidocaine was administered into the trachea using a mucosal atomisation device. Next, a gum elastic bougie was passed into the trachea, and the endotracheal tube 'railroaded' over the bougie. Intact neurology was confirmed by a brief neurological examination before the induction of general anaesthesia.

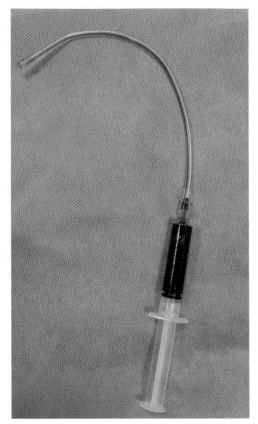

Figure 7.2. Mucosal atomisation device (MADgic®, Teleflex, Morrisville, USA).

How would you manage this case differently?

- Considering the ergonomics of awake tracheal intubation may reduce anxiety for some patients as they would be able to see less equipment. Having more equipment behind the patient and the operator standing in front of the patient may reduce anxiety. Constant verbal communication is essential to establish safe conscious sedation and to allay the patient's anxiety.

- Consideration of different sedative techniques could be used to make the procedure more comfortable for the patient; in this case a target-controlled infusion (TCI) of remifentanil was used. DAS guidelines also recommend adding in midazolam 0.5–1mg if there is a second anaesthetist present to monitor the patient. Table 7.1 shows alternative sedative drugs that may be used.

Table 7.1. Sedative drugs used for awake tracheal intubation*.

Agent	Dose	Maximum dose	Additional notes
Midazolam	30–50μg/kg	5mg (lower in older people)	
Fentanyl	0.5–1μg/kg	If used as a co-sedative 1.5μg/kg	
Remifentanil	TCI (Minto) effect site concentration 1–3ng/ml		May be used as a co-sedative with propofol or midazolam
Propofol	TCI effect site concentration of 0.5–1μg/ml		Best used with remifentanil Associated with the greatest risk of over-sedation as the sole agent
Dexmedetomidine	Bolus dose: 0.7–1μg/kg over 10 minutes Infusion: 0.3–0.7μg/kg/hour		

* Drug administration should be carefully titrated with close monitoring of sedation level.

- Awake tracheal intubation using videolaryngoscopy may offer a less stressful alternative to awake fibreoptic intubation for some patients.

Key points

- Awake tracheal intubation is considered an optimal technique of tracheal intubation in the presence of an unstable cervical spine.
- The use of a hyperangulated videolaryngoscope blade can provide a good view of the glottis with the patient's head and neck in a neutral position and cause minimal movement of the cervical spine.
- Good rapport with the patient and an appropriate explanation of the procedure may alleviate anxiety and increase the patient's compliance with the procedure, reduce the required depth of sedation and improve patient safety during the procedure.

References

1. Ahmad I, El-Boghdadly K, Bhagrath R, *et al*. Difficult Airway Society guidelines for awake tracheal intubation (ATI) in adults. *Anaesthesia* 2020; 75(4): 509-28.

2. Kramer A, Müller D, Pförtner R, *et al*. Fibreoptic vs videolaryngoscopic (C-MAC® D-BLADE) nasal awake intubation under local anaesthesia. *Anaesthesia* 2015; 70(4): 400-6.

3. Ramkumar V. Preparation of the patient and the airway for awake intubation. *Indian J Anaesth* 2011; 55(5): 442-7.

4. Vora J, Leslie D, Stacey M. Awake tracheal intubation. *BJA Educ* 2022; 22(8): 298-305.

Case scenario 8

Introduction

A 67-year-old woman presented for an elective total hip replacement with a background of rheumatoid arthritis.

Past medical history

- Rheumatoid arthritis, affecting most of her joints. She had sustained a previous subluxation of the atlantoaxial joint. This had required surgical decompression and fixation of the spine that was performed 7 years ago.
- A total knee replacement was performed 3 years ago under a technically difficult subarachnoid block.

Clinical examination

The patient was wheelchair bound due to severe arthritis and limited mobility.

She asked the anaesthetist to sit directly in front of her due to limited neck rotation. Her neck was fixed in a flexed position. Other airway examination findings included:

- Limited mouth opening with an inter-incisor distance of 2cm.
- Mallampati score 4.
- Severe kyphoscoliosis.
- BMI 22.8 (weight 55kg, height 155cm).

Investigations

A review of previous cervical spine X-rays showed occipital-cervical fusion (Figures 8.1 and 8.2). There were no further investigations available to evaluate the airway.

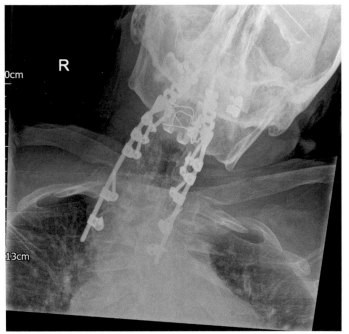

Figure 8.1. Anteroposterior view of cervical spine X-ray.

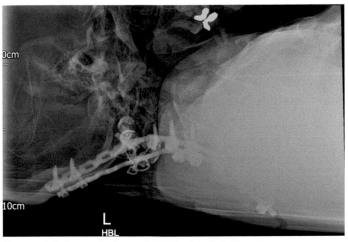

Figure 8.2. Lateral view of cervical spine X-ray.

How this case was managed

The two main options for anaesthetic management were general anaesthesia and central neuraxial block:

- Securing the airway in this patient would require awake tracheal intubation. In addition, with a fixed flexion of the cervical spine, there was a high chance of difficult bag valve mask ventilation. Rescue techniques such as a supraglottic airway device would probably also be difficult.

- Another option would be a central neuraxial block. The concern was, however, that it would be extremely difficult to secure the airway if there were any intra-operative complications. Furthermore, with the patient's short stature, there was a small but distinct possibility of a high spinal block. There was also a previous history of technical difficulty with a spinal anaesthetic. Therefore, the patient preferred general anaesthesia.

How was the airway managed in this patient?

Considering all these factors, the anaesthetist opted for general anaesthesia and awake fibreoptic intubation as the safest option for the patient. The procedure was explained to the patient and consent was taken. The plan was communicated during a team brief. The basic equipment required for awake fibreoptic intubation is shown in Figure 8.3.

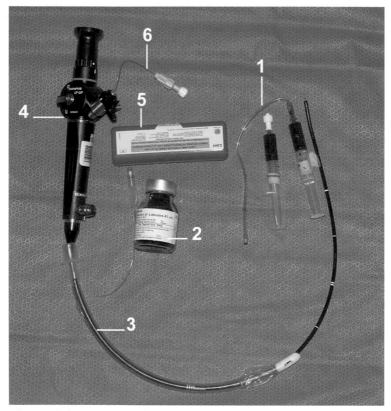

Figure 8.3. Drugs and equipment used for awake fibreoptic intubation. 1) Mucosal atomisation device. 2) 4% lidocaine. 3) Tracheal tube loaded on the fibreoptic scope. 4) Fibreoptic scope. 5) 5% lidocaine with 0.5% phenylephrine. 6) Epidural catheter.

Intubation strategy

Awake fibreoptic intubation via the oral route was planned. The procedure was performed by two experienced consultants. Adequate anaesthesia was achieved with 4% lidocaine, and a target-controlled infusion of remifentanil was used for conscious sedation. Despite this, the patient experienced gagging and coughing during the procedure. Awake intubation was completed via the oral route. Once the tracheal tube position was confirmed using capnography, a general anaesthetic was commenced.

The operation was successfully completed, and the patient was extubated at the end and transferred to the ward.

Postoperative review

The patient was reviewed on the first postoperative day. She had a full recollection of the events in the anaesthetic room and reported the experience as moderately unpleasant. She was given a full explanation of the events, the decision-making process and the need for awake intubation in her case. She found the conversation helpful and reassuring and had no further questions.

How would you manage this case differently?

- As per NAP5 findings, explicitly inform the patient of the risk of awareness in the context of difficult airway management. However, in this case, the patient was told about awake tracheal intubation.
- Pre-operative explanation of the technique and a patient leaflet giving details on why awake intubation is required and what to expect during the procedure are useful in reducing patient anxiety and improving patient satisfaction.
- Following topicalisation of the oropharynx, patients may experience difficulty in swallowing. Similarly, once the bronchoscope is advanced through the vocal cords, patients may experience a choking sensation. These problems should be explained to the patient.

- Consider using 10% lidocaine; this may provide a better quality topical anaesthesia of airway mucosa.
- Consider the use of sedative agents to allow for conscious sedation during the procedure.
- A high-flow nasal oxygenation device allows the delivery of warm, humidified oxygen at 30–70L/minute. It may also improve the quality of topical anaesthesia.
- Consideration of video-assisted fibreoptic intubation (VAFI) in which both flexible fibrescopes and videolaryngoscopes are used to improve the success rate of awake tracheal intubation.

Table 8.1. Local anaesthetic techniques for awake fibreoptic intubation via the nasal route.

Anatomy	Local anaesthetic drug	Total dose of local anaesthetic*
Nose	Co-phenylcaine (lidocaine 5% and phenylephrine 0.5%): 2ml	100mg
Pharynx	Lidocaine 4% administered through a 20G cannula connected to an oxygen flow at 3L/minute: 6ml	240mg
Larynx	Lidocaine 4% via an epidural catheter inserted via the suction port of the scope, 1ml above the vocal cords and 1ml below the vocal cords	80mg

* Total dose of local anaesthetic not to exceed >9mg/kg (lean body weight).

- Sedation using remifentanil TCI. Start with 1ng/ml and increase by 0.5ng/ml increments to a maximum of 3ng/ml.

Mackenzie technique of airway topicalisation

Oxygen tubing is connected to a peripheral venous catheter. The other end of the oxygen tubing is connected to an oxygen source, either an auxiliary oxygen flow meter of an anaesthetic machine or an oxygen cylinder. Oxygen flow is adjusted to 3–4L/minute. A 5ml syringe filled with local anaesthetic is connected to the injection port of the peripheral venous catheter (Figure 8.4).

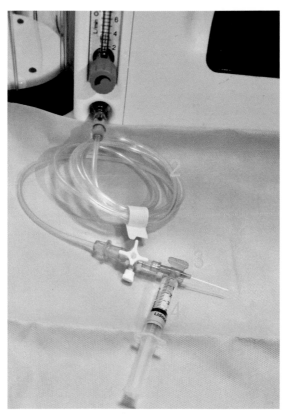

Figure 8.4. Set-up of the Mackenzie technique. 1) Oxygen source. 2) Oxygen tubing. 3) 20G cannula. 4) Syringe with lidocaine.

Local anaesthetic is slowly administered through the syringe (0.5ml at a time), producing a jet-like spray. Synchronisation of spray with each inspiration allows inhalation of droplets and topicalisation of the lower airway.

The DAS awake tracheal intubation guidelines suggest four steps for awake tracheal intubation:

1.   Oxygenate: it is recommended to start oxygenation early.
2.   Topicalise: lidocaine 10% spray can be used for the oropharynx, tonsillar pillars and base of the tongue (a total of 20–30 sprays synchronised with inspiration). One metered dose of spray delivers 10mg of lidocaine.
3.   Perform: this involves performing an endoscopy, preferably with the patient sitting up. It is important to consider the ergonomics (Figure 8.5) so that the operator can monitor the patient, see the monitor

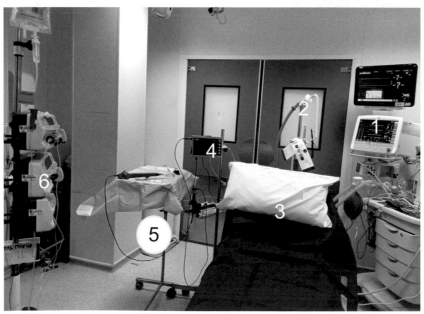

Figure 8.5. Ergonomics for the performance of awake fibreoptic intubation. 1) Patient monitor. 2) High-flow nasal oxygen device. 3) Patient. 4) Video monitor. 5) Operator. 6) Infusion pumps.

screen and maintain constant verbal communication with the patient. Patient cooperation is important, so that the patient can open their mouth and protrude their tongue to obtain a clear view of anatomical structures (Figure 8.6).

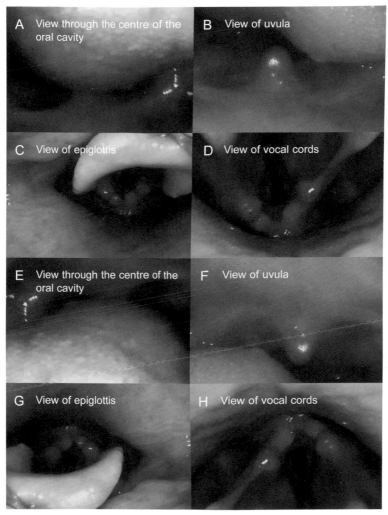

Figure 8.6. Endoscopic views obtained during oral fibreoptic intubation with the operator behind the patient (A-D) and the operator standing in front of the patient (E-H).

4.   Sedation with remifentanil alone is considered a safer option when only one operator is present. Additional drugs such as midazolam or propofol can be used if a second anaesthetist is present to administer drugs and monitor the patient.

Awake tracheal intubation is considered the gold standard for securing the airway in an anticipated difficult airway. However, there are certain limitations.

Awake intubation may not be possible in:

- Small children.
- Uncooperative patients, altered level of consciousness.
- Local anaesthetic sensitivity.
- Bleeding in the airway.

Key steps involved in performing awake fibreoptic intubation are:

- Patient preparation.
- Equipment preparation.
- Drugs preparation.
- Oxygenation.
- Monitoring.
- Local anaesthesia to the upper airway.
- Sedation.
- Endoscopy and local anaesthesia to the lower airway.
- 'Railroading' the tube.
- Checking the tube position: two-point confirmation.
- Securing the tube.
- Inducing general anaesthesia.

Key points

- The incidence of recall following awake fibreoptic intubation is higher when remifentanil is used for sedation as a sole agent, compared with propofol or benzodiazepine-based sedation, or a combination of two or more agents. However, a small number of patients may find the experience unpleasant despite sedation.
- The postoperative follow-up visit is important and serves two purposes. First, it gives the anaesthetist feedback on the effectiveness of the method of topicalisation and sedation used. But, more importantly, it is the time when questions can be answered, and reassurance and an explanation can be offered to the patient in cases where the effect of sedative medication is suboptimal.

References

1. Ahmad I, El-Boghdadly K, Bhagrath R, et al. Difficult Airway Society guidelines for awake tracheal intubation (ATI) in adults. *Anaesthesia* 2020; 75(4): 509-28.

2. Mackenzie I. A new method of drug application to the nasal passage. *Anaesthesia* 1998; 53(3): 309-10.

3. Mistry V, Tourville C, May M, et al. Comparison of patients' experience following awake and asleep fibreoptic intubation: a prospective observational study. *Trends Anaesth Crit Care* 2022; 42: 20-5.

4. Pandit J, Cook T, Shinde S, et al. AAGBI Guidelines, The "NAP5 Handbook": concise practice guidance on the prevention and management of accidental awareness during general anaesthesia; March 2019. Available from: https://www.nationalauditprojects.org.uk/the-NAP5-Handbook#pt.

5. Vora J, Leslie D, Stacey M. Awake tracheal intubation. *BJA Educ* 2022; 22(8): 298-305.

Case scenario 9

Introduction

A 74-year-old man with a base of tongue cancer and cervical lymphadenopathy presented for a tracheostomy, hemi-glossectomy, bilateral neck dissection and reconstruction with a left forearm free flap. The surgery was scheduled on a weekend elective operating list.

Past medical history

His coexisting medical conditions included:

- Obesity (BMI of 36kg/m^2).
- Hypertension, which was well controlled with medication.

Clinical examination

The anaesthetist reviewed the patient pre-operatively and performed a detailed airway assessment:

- There was a visible ulcerative lesion on the left side of the tongue.
- Mallampati score of 3.
- Mouth opening 3.8cm.
- Neck extension was limited.
- The thyromental distance measured 7cm.
- Neck circumference was 45cm.

Investigations

After examining the airway, the anaesthetist reviewed the results of previous investigations. An MRI scan of the head and neck showed an extensive left-sided tongue lesion measuring 5cm on the long axis. On the left side, the lesion encroached on the floor of the mouth.

How this case was managed

As it was a weekend, the remote-site endoscopy sterilisation room was closed. There was no reusable fibreoptic scope available on the day. A limited number of single-use scopes (Ambu® aScope™) were available, but they were reserved for use in airway emergencies.

The anaesthetist decided that awake tracheal intubation was the right choice for securing the airway. Due to the limited availability of fibreoptic scopes, he decided to perform an awake videolaryngoscopy with a hyperangulated blade as Plan A and video-assisted fibreoptic intubation as Plan B.

A remifentanil target-controlled infusion at 2–4ng/ml and 0.5mg of midazolam was used for sedation. The airway was anaesthetised in a manner used for performing awake fibreoptic intubation. Lidocaine, 4% solution, was applied to the oral cavity and the oropharynx using a McKenzie technique, as shown earlier in Figure 8.4. An oxygen flow of 3L/minute was used to atomise the local anaesthetic solution, injected through the port of the cannula.

An awake laryngoscopy was then performed with a C-MAC® videolaryngoscope hyperangulated blade (D-Blade). The best view obtained was 50% of the glottic opening seen on the videolaryngoscope monitor screen. The additional local anaesthetic solution was then applied to the epiglottis, the vocal cords and the trachea using a mucosal atomiser device (Figure 9.1).

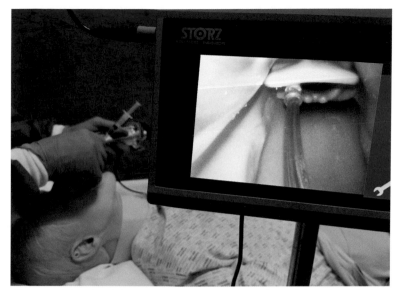

Figure 9.1. A video screen view showing lidocaine being administered using a mucosal atomisation device.

After adequate topical anaesthesia was achieved, the tracheal tube introducer (bougie) was inserted into the trachea, and a 7mm endotracheal tube was 'railroaded' over the bougie, its position in the trachea confirmed by the presence of a capnography trace and general anaesthesia was induced. The entire procedure was well tolerated by the patient.

How would you manage this case differently?

- This patient has clinical features suggesting difficult laryngoscopy and intubation. As this patient has a base of tongue lesion, fibreoptic intubation via the nasal route would be the author's most preferred option. A flexible nasal endoscopy in the anaesthetic room is useful in assessing the airway.
- During laryngoscopy, all precautions should be taken to avoid any trauma and bleeding from the tongue lesion; this will make further fibreoptic endoscopy more difficult.

- Awake videolaryngoscopy has become more popular due to increasing familiarity with videolaryngoscopes. This has been reflected in changes to difficult airway management algorithms to include awake videolaryngoscopy alongside awake fibreoptic intubations. In this case, a combined videolaryngoscope and fibrescope technique may also have been used.
- High-flow nasal oxygen could be used to reduce the risk of desaturation during awake intubation.
- Different methods exist to topicalise the upper airway for an awake technique, as described in Box 9.1. The Difficult Airway Society awake tracheal intubation guidelines recommend the use of 20–30 sprays of 10% lidocaine. Topicalisation using a mucosal atomisation device, McKenzie technique or 10% lidocaine spray are the most common methods for applying local anaesthetic to the upper airway. Spray-as-you-go techniques using an epidural catheter through the working channel of a fibreoptic scope or spray through a long mucosal atomisation device (for awake videolaryngoscopy) are the most commonly used methods.

Box 9.1. Different methods of topicalising the airway.

- Direct spray from a container of local anaesthetic.
- Ribbon gauze soaked in a local anaesthetic placed on the nasal cavity.
- McKenzie technique.
- Mucosal atomisation devices.
- Nebulisation of local anaesthetic.
- Spray-as-you-go technique.
- Regional anaesthesia with relevant nerve blocks.

Causes of potential difficult airways in patients with oral cancers

- Limitations on neck mobility.
- Limited mouth opening and jaw protrusion.
- Inability to protrude the tongue.
- Limited space within the upper airway due to the tumour, oedema or from previous surgery.
- Increased salivation.
- Potential for fixation of tissues due to tumour, previous radiotherapy or scarring from previous surgery.
- Increased risk of bleeding due to trauma to vascular tumours.
- Potential pre-existing airway compromise.

An awake intubation will be a primary plan for most. An experienced anaesthetist should be available to perform the procedure. If this is not an option, case postponement and front-of-neck access would be alternatives. Therefore, a head and neck surgeon should be immediately available to rescue failed awake intubation.

Key points

- Awake videolaryngoscopy has become a recognised alternative to awake fibreoptic intubations. With experience, the technique can be used in appropriately selected patients with an anticipated difficult airway.
- Ensure there is a plan made in case of a failed awake tracheal intubation, including the postponement of the case, high-risk general anaesthesia or front-of-neck access in the event a complete airway obstruction develops.

References

1. Ahmad I, El-Boghdadly K, Bhagrath R, *et al.* Difficult Airway Society guidelines for awake tracheal intubation (ATI) in adults. *Anaesthesia* 2020; 75(4): 509-28.

2. Kajekar P, Mendonca C, Danha R, Hillermann C. Awake tracheal intubation using Pentax Airway Scope in 30 patients: A Case series. *Indian J Anaesth* 2014; 58(4): 447-51.

3. Mendonca C, Mesbah A, Velayudhan A, Danha R. A randomised clinical trial comparing the flexible fibrescope and the Pentax Airway Scope (AWS)® for awake oral tracheal intubation. *Anaesthesia* 2016; 71(8): 908-14.

4. Mishra S, Bhatnagar S, Jha RR, Singhal AK. Airway management of patients undergoing oral cancer surgery: a retrospective study. *Eur J Anaesthesiol* 2005; 22(7): 510-4.

Case scenario 10

Introduction

A 34-year-old gentleman presented to the emergency department with a history of acute stridor. The ENT registrar had reviewed the patient and bleeped the ICU registrar to attend due to concerns about his clinical presentation and the potential need to secure the patient's airway. He had been moved into the resuscitation area for closer monitoring. On further questioning, the patient reported a 3-day history of sore throat with associated voice change and loss of appetite. He also had difficulty swallowing and was finding it difficult to lie flat.

Past medical history

He had no other past medical history to note.

Clinical examination

From the end of the bed, the patient was noted to be sitting up, was unable to swallow his secretions, and had tissues in his hand from wiping his saliva.

His observations showed:

- Oxygen saturation of 98% with an adrenaline nebuliser ongoing.
- Respiratory rate of 20 breaths/minute.
- Haemodynamically stable.

There was no evidence of respiratory distress and on disconnecting the adrenaline nebuliser there was no audible stridor.

An airway assessment revealed:

- Full range of movements of the neck.
- Mallampati was thought to be 3, although this view was impaired due to pooling of secretions.
- Mouth opening was greater than three fingers' breadth.
- At this point, the patient had received intravenous antibiotics, dexamethasone and analgesia. He had received nebulised bronchodilators and was on his second nebulised adrenaline.

Investigations

Blood tests were taken and their results were pending. A nasendoscopy was performed by the ENT registrar: there was evidence of a swollen epiglottis; however, the glottic inlet could not be visualised due to gross swelling in the supraglottic area.

How this case was managed

A decision was made to definitively secure the patient's airway in theatre following a discussion with the ENT registrar. The anaesthetic consultant was contacted for airway support, with a level 3 ICU bed arranged for ongoing support. The ENT consultant was asked to attend theatre, and the patient's relatives were updated on the airway plan.

What are your concerns about the case?

- Potential deterioration of airway over time.
- Nasendoscopy failed to visualise the glottic inlet.
- Loss of airway during airway manipulation.
- High-stress scenario with human factors at play.
- Need for quick decision making.
- The anaesthetist's own experience and skill level.

What are the options to secure this patient's airway?

The following plans were discussed with the patient and his family:

- High-risk general anaesthesia induction.
- An awake fibreoptic intubation.
- Gas induction.
- Emergency tracheostomy.

Airway management

The patient was transferred to the anaesthetic room with full monitoring on a FiO_2 of 100% via a 15L/minute non-rebreathe mask. The patient's oxygen saturation remained at 100% throughout the transfer.

An airway team was arranged that included two consultant anaesthetists (one who had an interest in difficult airway management), 2 ODPs, 1 ODP in training, an ICU registrar (anaesthetist in training) and the ENT consultant.

An initial airway plan was made for an intravenous induction with remifentanil, propofol and rocuronium. Sugammadex was available for emergency reversal. Plan A was to use a C-MAC® D-Blade videolaryngoscope to facilitate oral intubation and rescue using a fibreoptic scope. Plan B was a surgeon performing front-of-neck access. Equipment was kept on standby. The ENT consultant was on standby to perform front-of-neck access first and then to convert it to a formal tracheostomy.

On further review of the patient in the anaesthetic room, the patient remained haemodynamically stable, and oxygen saturations remained stable at 100%. The airway plan was changed, and a decision was made to anaesthetise the patient for awake fibreoptic intubation. He was positioned at approximately 45° sitting up, and high-flow nasal oxygen was commenced (as shown in Figure 11.2) with full monitoring *in situ*. Visualisation of the glottic inlet with a fibreoptic bronchoscope via the oral route was unsuccessful by both the anaesthetic and ENT consultant.

How this scenario was managed

Awake nasal intubation was attempted following nasal topicalisation with 5% lidocaine and 0.5% phenylephrine spray. A size 6mm ID tracheal tube was preloaded onto a fibreoptic scope and inserted through the left nostril. There was difficulty in visualising structures; however, air bubbles were visible. As the fibreoptic scope was advanced further, the scope was found to be in the trachea. A nasal tube was easily advanced into the trachea. However, as the patient was likely to require prolonged ventilatory support, an oral tube was preferable.

What was the next step?

In this case, an epidural catheter was passed through the suction catheter of the fibreoptic scope, and the trachea was anaesthetised. The nasal tracheal tube was then advanced, and inflated, and its position was

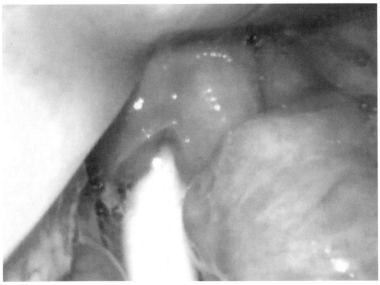

Figure 10.1. View of the nasal tracheal tube *in situ*.

confirmed using end-tidal capnography. Propofol was started to sedate the patient, and rocuronium was given to provide muscle paralysis. A plan was then made to convert the nasal to an oral tracheal tube using a video-assisted fibreoptic intubation (VAFI) technique. The videolaryngoscope (C-MAC® D-Blade) was used to visualise the glottic inlet (Figure 10.1). The fibreoptic scope loaded with a size 7mm ID tracheal tube was advanced toward the glottic inlet. Once in position, the nasal tracheal tube cuff was deflated to allow passage of the fibreoptic scope alongside the nasal tube. Once the trachea was visualised, the nasal tube was gently withdrawn, and the fibreoptic scope was advanced to visualise the carina. At this point, the nasal tube was fully withdrawn, and the oral tube was 'railroaded' over the fibreoptic scope into the trachea (Figure 10.2). Correct placement in the trachea was confirmed using a fibreoptic scope and capnography.

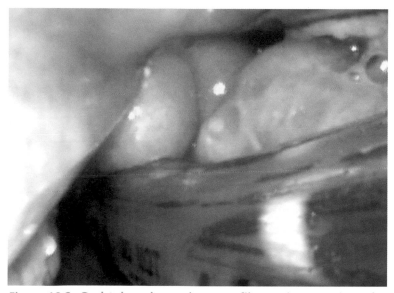

Figure 10.2. Oral tube advanced over a fibreoptic scope into the trachea (fibreoptic scope and oral tube both *in situ* in the image).

Post-intubation

The patient was subsequently transferred to an ICU, where he completed a course of steroids and antibiotics with regular ENT reviews and input. Daily sedation holds were performed with assessments of a cuff leak. The patient was successfully extubated a few days later. There were no airway complications or adverse events.

How would you manage this case differently?

- In difficult airway case management, clear communication between team members on the airway plan provides a reduction in adverse human factors, improving the success of the team.
- It is important to give a clear briefing to the team and pre-delegate roles to each team member.
- It is safer to perform the procedure in the operating theatre to allow greater space and the presence of a scrub team alongside the ENT surgeon if there is the need to perform an emergency front-of-neck access and tracheostomy.
- In a situation in which a patient is tired, drowsy and uncooperative for awake intubation, high-risk general anaesthesia and front-of-neck access may be the only option available to secure the airway.

Nasal versus oral tracheal tube in critical care

Fibrescopes can be used to facilitate tracheal intubation by either the nasal or oral route and form a cornerstone of difficult airway management worldwide. It is a useful technique allowing a secure airway to be established before the onset of general anaesthesia. It involves several different techniques to ensure success from a cooperative patient, adequate airway topicalisation and being able to identify anatomy through skilful scope handling.

As highlighted in this case, having a nasal tracheal tube may not be the most suitable route of intubation for a prolonged period. Due to the narrow lumen of the nasal tube required to pass through the nares, passing a suction catheter may be difficult both due to lumen size and also the length of standard suction catheters. This may increase the risk of developing ventilator-acquired pneumonia. There may be less familiarity with nasal tubes among staff, increasing the risk of displacement or unintentional extubation. Pressure sores may also develop at the nares due to the weight of the ventilator circuit over a prolonged period of time on a relatively vulnerable small area leading to increased morbidity for the patient.

Differences between nasal and oral fibreoptic intubations include:

- It is anatomically more favourable to use the nasal route to view the laryngeal inlet as the scope passes from the nasopharynx to the posterior oropharynx in the midline (Figures 10.3 and 10.4).
- The nasal route may be a more suitable route for patients with limited mouth opening, an enlarged tongue, and a base of tongue malignancy.
- The nasal route may provide better surgical access for intraoral procedures.

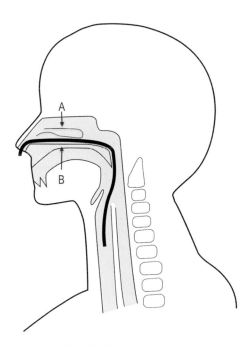

Figure 10.3. Route followed by the fibreoptic scope during nasal intubation. A) Inferior turbinate. B) Hard palate.

- Need to use vasoconstrictors to minimise the risk of bleeding from the nasal mucosa.
- There is a risk of nosebleeds due to trauma on passage of the fibreoptic scope or tracheal tube.

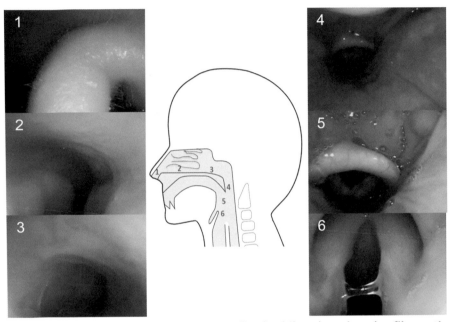

Figure 10.4. Anatomical structures visualised while advancing the fibreoptic scope through the nasal route. 1) Fibreoptic scope entering the nostril. 2) Fibreoptic scope at the anterior part of the nostril (view of inferior turbinate). 3) View of the posterior nasal aperture (choana). 4) Distant view of the epiglottis from the nasopharynx. 5) Closer view of the epiglottis from the laryngopharynx. 6) Fibreoptic scope passing through the glottic inlet.

Awake fibreoptic intubation

The key steps involved in awake fibreoptic intubation are described in Figure 10.5.

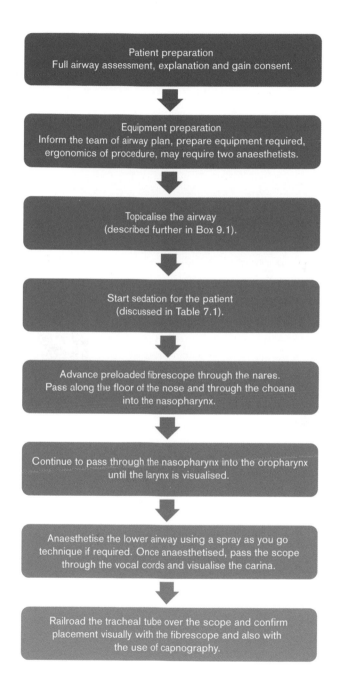

Figure 10.5. Flow diagram of the key steps in awake fibreoptic intubation.

Key points

- An awake tracheal intubation remains the gold standard method of managing an anticipated difficult tracheal intubation or difficult face mask ventilation.
- This case highlights the use of high-flow nasal oxygen to facilitate pre-oxygenation of the patient and prolong the apnoea time. This may be more relevant in critically ill patients with higher oxygen demand.
- A combined VAFI technique improves the success rate of tracheal intubation and tube exchange from the nasal to the oral route.

References

1. Ahmad I, El-Boghdadly K, Bhagrath R, *et al*. Difficult Airway Society guidelines for awake tracheal intubation (ATI) in adults. *Anaesthesia* 2020; 75(4): 509-28.
2. Chauhan V, Acharya G. Nasal intubation: a comprehensive review. *Indian J Crit Care Med* 2016; 20(11): 662-7.
3. Collins SR, Blank RS. Fiberoptic intubation: an overview and update. *Respir Care* 2014; 59(6): 865-78; discussion 878.

Case scenario 11

Introduction

An 86-year-old female patient presented for an urgent panendoscopy and biopsy of a pharyngeal lesion. She had been experiencing dysphagia over the preceding weeks before admission. The dysphagia was due to the ingestion of solid foods with the symptoms progressively worsening, to the point her diet consisted mainly of ice cream and tea.

On further questioning she denied any positional dyspnoea, stridor or any other breathing difficulties. However, she admitted having to suddenly pause for breath while walking, as she had a sensation of something being stuck in her throat.

Past medical history

- Hypertension, treated with antihypertensive agents. Pre-operatively, her blood pressure was well controlled.
- History of a thyroid nodule that had no surgical input to date.
- Osteoarthritis, resulting in a limitation of her mobility.

Clinical examination

A thorough airway examination was performed and she was found to have:

- Mallampati class 2.
- Inter-incisor distance of 3.5cm.
- A good ability to flex the neck but limited neck extension.
- No goitre or palpable masses in the neck.

Investigations

A review of the clinical records informed that a flexible nasendoscopy had been performed 3 days before and showed a mass lesion in the supraglottic area. The captured image is shown in Figure 11.1.

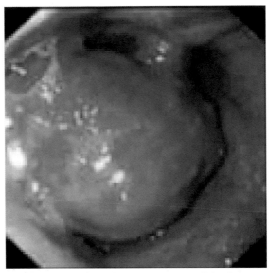

Figure 11.1. Nasoendoscopy view of the lesion.

How this case was managed

The anaesthetist discussed the case with the surgeon. The consultant surgeon felt that the lesion was most likely to be a laryngeal cyst and that it would reduce in size following needle aspiration. While performing nasendoscopy, the surgeon was briefly able to visualise the anterior commissure. The airway management plans were as follows:

- Taking into consideration the fact that the patient had significant airway pathology, the options considered were an awake tracheal intubation or awake tracheostomy.

- As the patient did not have any signs of respiratory distress, an awake fibreoptic intubation was chosen as Plan A.
- Plan B was a tracheostomy performed under local anaesthetic and conscious sedation.

Intubation strategy

An awake tracheal intubation was successfully performed via the nasal route using a flexible bronchoscope.

The patient was sedated with fentanyl 50μg, midazolam 0.5mg and a target-controlled infusion of propofol at 0.6μg/ml, ensuring the patient was conscious and responsive to commands.

Bypassing the mass and visualising the vocal cords with the fibreoptic scope required considerable skill. Manoeuvres such as asking the patient to attempt phonation and sniffing had no effect. By asking the patient to take a deep inhalation, the vocal cords were then visualised, and the flexible bronchoscope was passed into the trachea. A size 6mm ID microlaryngeal tube was 'railroaded' over the flexible bronchoscope.

When attempting to 'railroad' the endotracheal tube over the bronchoscope, an obstruction was encountered that was overcome by rotating the tube in an anticlockwise direction.

Correct placement of the tracheal tube was confirmed by visualising the carina and the presence of end-tidal carbon dioxide ($ETCO_2$).

Intra-operative findings

During rigid laryngoscopy, the surgeon found that the mass was located posteriorly, above (proximal to) the vocal cords and was originating from one of the arytenoid cartilages and was solid rather than cystic in nature, and the vocal cords were intact. Biopsies were taken to guide further management. The histology was reported as soft tissue sarcoma.

Extubation strategy

The anaesthetist was reluctant to extubate this patient's trachea.

Although the vocal cords were fully visible during the surgical procedure, it was felt this was due to the effect of the endotracheal tube displacing the mass posteriorly. There was concern that if the tube was removed, the mass would move back into its original position above the vocal cords.

Due to the intra-operative biopsy, there was an increased risk of intraluminal oedema. Although the patient had no breathing difficulties before the procedure, a further narrowing of the patient's airway may have led to respiratory distress.

When considering potential rescue techniques, blood present in the pharynx would make a repeat fibreoptic intubation even more challenging if any problems occurred.

The surgeon agreed to perform a tracheostomy that was technically challenging due to the limited extension of the neck and a deviated trachea.

How would you manage this case differently?

- High-flow nasal oxygen (Figure 11.2) could be used to both pre-oxygenate the patient and provide apnoeic ventilation during a potentially difficult intubation.

  The nasal Optiflow™ system comprises a humidification unit containing a flow driver and humidifier. This connects to a standard pipeline oxygen supply and delivers humidified, warm oxygen to the patient through modified tubing and nasal prongs. This gives the advantage of pre-oxygenation while leaving the oropharynx clear for either anaesthetic or surgical access. It produces turbulent flow within the oropharynx, replenishing oxygen supplies and avoiding entrainment of air. This results in oxygenation through the passive mechanism of the aventilatory mass flow. High flow also creates a CPAP effect up to 5cmH$_2$O. It reduces anatomical dead space and leads to some degree of carbon dioxide clearance.

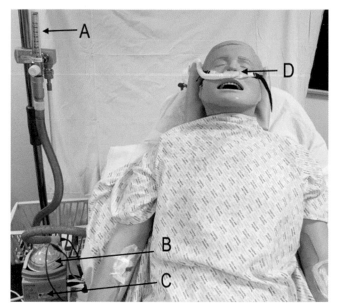

Figure 11.2. Optiflow™ high-flow nasal oxygen delivery system. A) Flow meter. B) Humidifier pot. C) Temperature control unit. D) Nasal prongs.

Common pitfalls with the technique come from inexperienced users either not being able to set up the kit or not having the kit available. Bleeding within the oropharynx is a relative contraindication due to the aerosolisation of the blood. A patent airway is essential to allow successful oxygenation during the period of apnoea. The presence of a patent airway maintains a continuous column of oxygen from the upper airway to the alveoli.

- The ENT surgeon should be present and scrubbed to aid with front-of-neck access (FONA) if a 'cannot intubate cannot oxygenate' situation arises. Equipment required for FONA should be readily available. All staff should be familiar with the equipment required for front-of-neck access.

- Ultrasound can be used to identify and mark the cricothyroid membrane (Figure 11.3), especially in a deviated trachea. This is important if front-of-neck access or a tracheostomy was required.

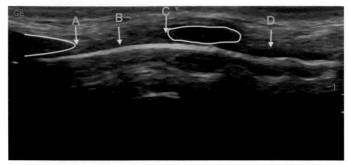

Figure 11.3. Ultrasound image of the cricothyroid membrane; longitudinal view. A) Caudal end of the thyroid cartilage. B) Midpoint of the cricothyroid membrane. C) Cephalad end of the cricoid cartilage. D) First tracheal ring.

- A well planned extubation strategy and an assessment of the need for the high dependency unit postoperatively could have been arranged as part of a multidisciplinary team (MDT) discussion before the procedure.

Methods to optimise intubation during awake fibreoptic intubation via the oral route

- The use of oral intubating airways (route guides) to guide the fibreoptic bronchoscope (Figure 11.4). The most commonly used devices include a William's airway, Ovassapian airway, Berman intubating airway and bronchoscope airway. These ensure that the bronchoscope is maintained in the centre of the oropharynx.
- Asking an assistant to provide a jaw thrust, asking the patient to phonate and asking the patient to protrude their tongue. These manoeuvres will open the airway giving more space to advance the bronchoscope.
- Always ensure that the bronchoscope is in the midline and identify an anatomical structure and keep the target structure in the centre of the field.
- Use oral suction to clear the secretions and maintain a good view.

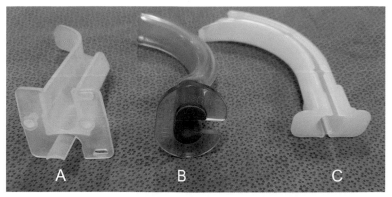

Figure 11.4. Oral intubating airway used in clinical practice to improve the success of oral fibreoptic intubation. A) Bronchoscope airway. B) Modified Guedel airway. C) Berman airway.

- The tube is likely to impinge at the arytenoids and aryepiglottic folds (Figure 11.5). Preloading the tube so that the bevel faces backward, or withdrawal and anticlockwise rotation, can overcome this problem.

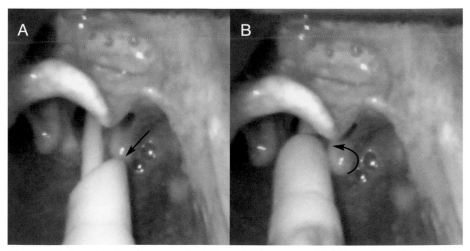

Figure 11.5. Tube impingement at the right arytenoid (A) and anticlockwise rotation (B).

- Tube tip design and tube size are other factors that lead to successful awake fibreoptic intubation (Figures 11.6 and 11.7). The larger the

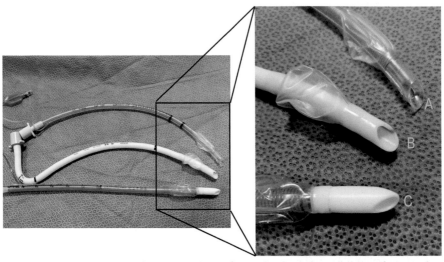

Figure 11.6. Tip design of various tubes. A) Standard reinforced tube. B) Portex® nasal tube. C) Single-use intubating laryngeal mask airway (ILMA) tube.

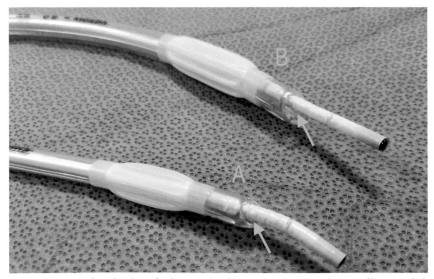

Figure 11.7. Tube size in relation to the fibreoptic scope. The smaller gap (A) and larger gap (B) between the fibreoptic bronchoscope and the tracheal tube are due to the size difference in the tracheal tube.

tube size in relation to the diameter of the fibreoptic bronchoscope, the higher the risk of impingement. Tracheal tubes with shorter bevels and soft silicone tips (for example, the intubating LMA tube) facilitate 'railroading' the tube over the fibreoptic bronchoscope and minimise tube impingement.

Key points

- The airway evaluation must include an assessment for ease of front-of-neck access. This can involve the use of ultrasonography.
- High-flow nasal oxygenation may be used in patients with a potentially difficult intubation to allow good pre-oxygenation and apnoeic ventilation.
- Patients with an anticipated difficult airway should have a well planned extubation strategy.

References

1. Collins SR, Blank RS. Fibreoptic Intubation: an overview and update. *Respir Care* 2014; 59(6): 865-78; discussion 878.

2. Difficult Airway Society Extubation Guidelines Group, Popat M, Mitchell V, *et al.* Difficult Airway Society guidelines for the management of tracheal extubation. *Anaesthesia* 2012; 67(3): 318-40.

3. Fisher & Paykel Healthcare. Optiflow™ nasal high flow therapy. Available from: https://www.fphcare.com/en-gb/hospital/adult-respiratory/optiflow/.

4. Greer JR, Smith SP, Strang T. A comparison of tracheal tube tip designs on the passage of an endotracheal tube during oral fiberoptic intubation. *Anesthesiology* 2001; 94(5): 729-31; discussion 5A.

5. Patel A, Nouraei SAR. Transnasal Humidified Rapid-Insufflation Ventilatory Exchange (THRIVE): a physiological method of increasing apnoea time in patients with difficult airways. *Anaesthesia* 2015; 70(3): 323-9.

6. Rai Y, You-Ten E, Zasso F, *et al.* The role of ultrasound in front-of-neck access for cricothyroid membrane identification: a systematic review. *J Crit Care* 2020; 60: 161-8.

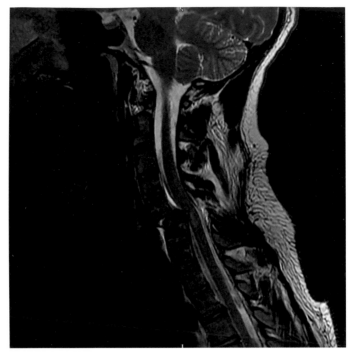

Figure 12.1. MRI cervical spine.

Pre-operative management

A review of the medical records revealed that the first attempt at stabilisation using an anterior approach (anterior cervical decompression and fusion) was undertaken 3 days before, shortly after admission. At the time, the airway was secured using awake fibreoptic intubation via the nasal route. Sedation was administered using a target-controlled infusion of propofol and remifentanil. A tracheal tube of 6mm internal diameter (LMA® Fastrach™ ETT, Teleflex Medical, Ireland) was easily passed through the nose into the trachea, and the tip visualised 3cm above the carina.

The entire procedure was uneventful and no problems were encountered during the course of the anaesthetic. Unfortunately, the surgeon was unable to complete the procedure using an anterior approach. The patient was extubated awake, cervical traction was applied, and a second procedure using a combined posterior and anterior approach was scheduled.

How this case was managed

The anaesthetist decided to perform awake fibreoptic intubation using the nasal route and the same type of tracheal tube.

Intubation strategy

The awake tracheal intubation procedure was uneventful and well tolerated with cervical traction *in situ*. Following the evaluation of neurological function, general anaesthesia was induced and the patient turned to a prone position. A few minutes later it was noticed that the bellows of the ventilator were not filling up and a low tidal volume alarm was activated. When the fresh gas flow was increased, an audible air leak was noted. Approximately 200ml of the fresh gas flow was lost with each breath. The leak persisted after the patient was turned back to the supine position.

What was the next step in managing this patient's airway?

The manual in-line stabilisation of the head was maintained, and the help of a consultant experienced in difficult airway management was requested. Ventilation was continued using 100% oxygen and high fresh gas flow. The consultant experienced in difficult airway management performed an indirect videolaryngoscopy using a GlideScope® videolaryngoscope. The endotracheal tube cuff was visualised at the level of the vocal cords, along with a significant amount of blood in the oropharynx. It was not possible to advance the tube further into the trachea without the aid of a bougie or a fibreoptic scope. It was difficult to pass the bougie through the size 6mm ID nasal tube.

What was the next step?

A stop-and-think action was taken and the team discussed the available options. The surgeon mentioned that the duration of surgery was likely to be more than 6 hours. The anaesthetist decided that it was easier to use a size 7mm ID oral tube to facilitate prolonged ventilation during the intra-operative period and, if required, during the postoperative period.

A video-assisted oral fibreoptic intubation using a combination of GlideScope® and fibreoptic bronchoscope was planned. The fibreoptic bronchoscope was loaded with a 7mm ID reinforced oral tracheal tube. As there was a considerable amount of oropharyngeal bleeding, the consultant utilised an indirect view on the GlideScope® monitor to insert the fibreoptic bronchoscope orally (Figure 12.2), through the vocal cords, past the endotracheal tube (ETT) cuff and into the trachea. The correct placement of the bronchoscope in the trachea was confirmed by visualising the carina. The nasal ETT was then removed, and the oral ETT 'railroaded' over the fibreoptic bronchoscope. The position of the tube in the trachea was then confirmed

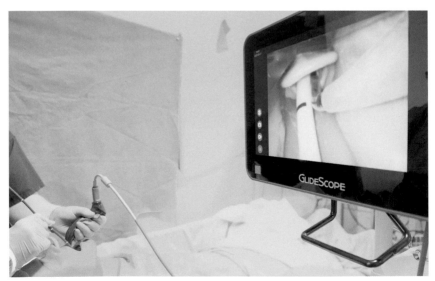

Figure 12.2. Indirect view using GlideScope® showing a fibreoptic scope passed orally beyond the vocal cords.

with the bronchoscope, and the presence of $EtCO_2$. The endotracheal tube was then secured in position, and the patient was repositioned.

How would you manage this case differently?

- Awake tracheal intubation to secure the airway via the oral route using a videolaryngoscope could have been considered as the primary airway plan.
- Video-assisted fibreoptic intubation via the oral route would require two anaesthetists present, one to perform videolaryngoscopy and one to drive the fibreoptic scope.
- It is important to ensure that the tube is well secured before placing the patient in a prone position. Having an awareness of the position the surgical team requires the patient to be in may assist in determining how the tube is secured. For this procedure the patient was required to be in a prone position with the head clamped using Mayfield® skull pins, as shown in Figure 12.3.

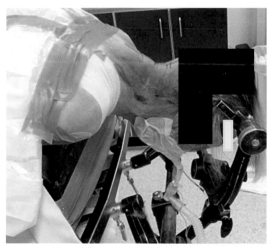

Figure 12.3. Patient in a prone position, head fixed on a Mayfield® skull clamp. The tracheal tube is firmly secured using adhesive tape.

- Always have a management strategy if the tube displaces or accidental extubation happens in the prone position.
- In the event an airway crisis happens in the prone position, additional staff and equipment are required to turn the patient to a supine position.
- Consider pre-allocating roles to team members to mitigate the risks of accidental extubation or if tube displacement occurs. For example, team member A is allocated the task of getting the trolley to turn the patient supine, team member B is allocated the task of setting up the fibreoptic scope, etc.).

What are the potential causes of low tidal volumes?

The potential causes are explored in Box 12.1 below. These can be split into patient, environmental and surgical factors.

Box 12.1. Causes of low tidal volumes.

Patient factors	Equipment factors	Surgical factors

• Ventilator dysynchrony:
  - inadequate muscle relaxation;
  - light plane of sedation.
• Pneumothorax.
• Bronchospasm/ laryngospasm.
	• Leak in the circuit.
	• Disconnection.
	• Poor seal on supraglottic airway device.
	• Deflated cuff on tracheal tube.
	• Damaged pilot balloon.
	• Malpositioned tracheal tube.
		• Pneumoperitoneum.
		• External compression on chest wall.
		• Breech of pleural cavity.

How would you troubleshoot a low tidal volume alarm to diagnose the cause?

The flow chart below (Figure 12.4) gives a systematic way to troubleshoot a low tidal volume alarm on a ventilator. If at any stage there are concerns, call for help at the earliest opportunity.

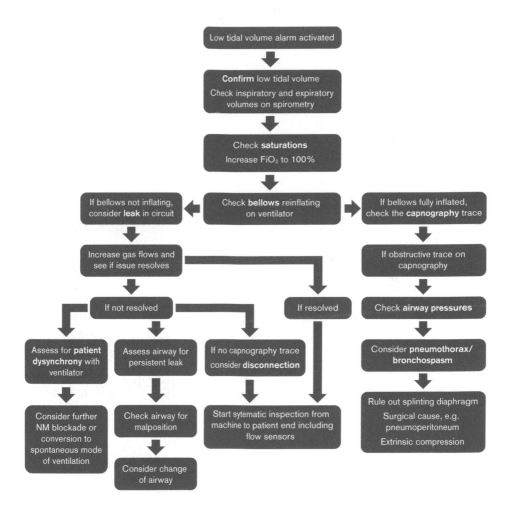

Figure 12.4. Management of a low tidal volume alarm.

Key points

- Although awake fibreoptic intubation is technically easier to perform via a nasal route, this route is not appropriate for all surgical procedures. The length of the nasal tube must be adequate to ensure the tracheal tube cuff is safely placed below the level of the vocal cords. In this case, the tracheal tube used for the nasal route was relatively shorter, as just a 2cm outward movement when moved into a prone position resulted in displacement of the tube and an airway emergency.

- Equipment and additional help are required to manage this crisis effectively. Therefore, pre-delegation of roles and mention of a management strategy for accidental tube displacement at the team briefing is useful for shared decision making.

- In an emergency, as soon as the patient is stabilised, a stop-and-think moment will enable you to choose the best option.

References

1. Alhomary M, Ramadan E, Curran E, Walsh SR. Videolaryngoscopy vs. fibreoptic bronchoscopy for awake tracheal intubation: a systematic review and meta-analysis. *Anaesthesia* 2018; 73(9): 1151-61.

2. Desai N, Ratnayake G, Onwochei DN, *et al.* Airway devices for awake tracheal intubation in adults: a systematic review and network meta-analysis. *Br J Anaesth* 2021; 127(4): 636-47.

Case scenario 13

Introduction

A 79-year-old man was scheduled to undergo an elective right total nephrectomy for a large renal tumour.

Past medical history

- Ankylosing spondylitis, long-standing.
- Restrictive lung disease.
- Atrial fibrillation.
- Previous lumbar spinal fusion.

Clinical examination

The patient was reviewed within the pre-operative assessment clinic. Given the long history of ankylosing spondylitis, the anaesthetist performed a thorough airway assessment:

- Inter-incisor distance was 4.5cm.
- Mallampati grade was 2.
- Neck extension was not possible.

Functionally he reported that he was unable to manage a full flight of stairs due to a combination of poor mobility and shortness of breath; however, he had mobilised >50m to the clinic on level ground.

The patient reported no problems with previous anaesthetics. The anaesthetist carefully reviewed the previous anaesthetic records and found that the patient had undergone two minor surgical procedures 3 years ago.

In both cases, the bag valve mask ventilation was documented as easy, as was the insertion of the supraglottic airway and ventilation through the device. Based on his past medical history, echocardiography and pulmonary function tests were arranged.

Investigations

His echocardiogram showed a left ventricular ejection fraction of 55% (normal ejection fraction between 50–70%) and a pulmonary artery pressure of 49mmHg (normal pulmonary artery systolic pressure 18–25mmHg). His spirometry confirmed a mild restrictive disorder.

How this case was managed

An awake fibreoptic intubation via the oral route was planned. After explaining the procedure to the patient, he firmly declined, on the grounds of no problems with past anaesthetics. Therefore, a decision was made for asleep fibreoptic intubation as in Plan B.

Intubation strategy

Intravenous induction of anaesthesia was followed by neuromuscular blockade achieved with rocuronium. The bag valve mask ventilation was easy. Oral fibreoptic-guided intubation was attempted, but the anaesthetist was unable to visualise the vocal cords with the fibreoptic bronchoscope. The epiglottis was visible, yet it was impossible to negotiate the fibreoptic bronchoscope beyond the epiglottis.

What was the next step?

Help was summoned from a consultant with a special interest in difficult airway management. He performed videolaryngoscopy with a channelled King Vision™ laryngoscope. With this technique, 50% of the glottic opening was visible. However, when the passage of the endotracheal tube was attempted, it repeatedly hit the arytenoid cartilage. Manoeuvres to manipulate the airway were attempted, including slight withdrawal and rotation of the tracheal tube with no effect. It was not possible to advance the tube into the trachea.

How was the patient intubated?

The fibreoptic bronchoscope was inserted through the tracheal tube, which, in turn, was loaded into the channelled blade of the King Vision™ videolaryngoscope (Figures 13.1 and 13.2). The bronchoscope was then advanced into the trachea, guided by the view on the King Vision™ monitor. After the scope was successfully placed in the trachea, the tracheal tube was advanced over the bronchoscope, past the vocal cords.

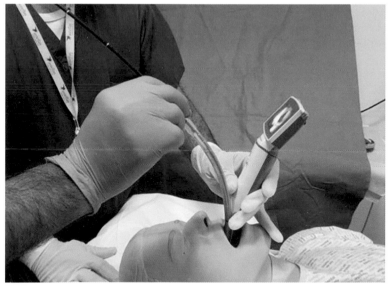

Figure 13.1. Combined videolaryngoscopy and fibreoptic bronchoscopy technique.

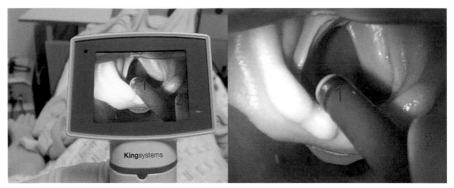

Figure 13.2. Views obtained using a videolaryngoscope monitor. 1) Tip of the fibreoptic bronchoscope. 2) Tip of the tracheal tube.

Intra-operative management

After securing the airway, the anaesthetist attempted to insert an epidural catheter for postoperative pain relief. Due to technical difficulties, this failed and an intrathecal injection of morphine was performed for postoperative pain relief.

The surgeon experienced serious technical difficulties with the procedure, and the nephrectomy was eventually abandoned. The total surgical time was 8.5 hours. There was significant blood loss associated with a massive transfusion. At the end of the surgery, the patient had a haemoglobin concentration of 8.8g/L. Blood gas analysis demonstrated metabolic acidosis (pH 7.23, a base deficit of 6.7mEq/L and lactate of 4.7mmol/L). Adequate oxygenation was achieved with the inspired oxygen concentration of 40%.

Postoperative management

There was a concern about the patient developing hypoxaemia in the postoperative period in the face of difficult intubation. The patient was transferred to the intensive care unit and ventilated, with a plan for delayed extubation.

Before the extubation, an airway exchange catheter was inserted (as shown in Figure 14.1), and awake extubation was performed by an anaesthetist experienced in the technique. The catheter was left *in situ* and remained well tolerated by the patient. It was removed 24 hours later when he was able to vocalise and cough well. Details on practical aspects of inserting airway exchange catheters are described in Case scenario 14.

How would you manage this case differently?

- In an anticipated difficult airway, the awake technique is the gold standard for managing the airway. The patient should be provided with adequate information on the benefits of the awake technique and the consequences of failed intubation.
- Following the initial failure at tracheal intubation, a careful decision should be taken whether to proceed to Plan B of the Difficult Airway Society guidelines of managing unanticipated difficult intubation.
- The option to wake up the patient to perform awake tracheal intubation at a later stage can be considered in all elective situations.
- Ensure good communication with the patient to highlight the risks of management of a difficult airway, including that conditions may have changed in comparison with his previous anaesthetics.

Key points

- Videolaryngoscopes usually provide an excellent view of the vocal cords. Obtaining a good view does not, however, guarantee easy intubation.
- Depending on the type of videolaryngoscope, withdrawal of the videolaryngoscope to obtain a partial view of the larynx, use of a bougie, changing the size of the laryngoscope blade or the tracheal tube, or use of tubes that can be flexed dynamically during intubation may provide a solution.
- A fibreoptic bronchoscope should be used in combination with a videolaryngoscope, as described in this scenario, to improve the success rate of tracheal intubation.

References

1.   Frerk C, Mitchell VS, McNarry AF, *et al.* Difficult Airway Society 2015 guidelines for management of unanticipated difficult intubation in adults. *Br J Anaesth* 2015; 115(6): 827-48.

2.   Gupta A, Kapoor D, Awana M, Lehl G. Fiberscope assisted videolaryngoscope intubation in the surgical treatment of TMJ ankylosis. *J Maxillofac Oral Surg* 2015; 14(2): 484-6.

3.   Leslie D, Stacey M. Awake intubation. *Contin Educ Anaesth Crit Care Pain* 2015; 15(2): 64-7.

4.   Niforopoulou P, Pantazopoulos I, Demestiha T, *et al.* Videolaryngoscopes in the adult airway management: a topical review of the literature. *Acta Anaesthesiol Scand* 2010; 54(9): 1050-61.

Case scenario 14

Introduction

A 51-year-old woman was scheduled to undergo an urgent mitral valve replacement due to severe, symptomatic mitral stenosis. Her symptoms had been rapidly progressing in the weeks before her admission, and she now had dyspnoea at rest and marked ascites.

Past medical history

- Prosthetic aortic valve.
- A cardiac pacemaker.
- Von Willebrand disease.
- She had a long history of cervical spine disease.

On further questioning she revealed that at the age of 48 she suffered a fall and sustained a cervical spine injury leading to hemiparesis and a phrenic nerve injury. At the time, urgent surgical stabilisation of her cervical spine was necessary, and she was ventilated in intensive care for 16 weeks following the event. Finally, 6 months before the admission, she underwent an elective fixation of the cervical spine with fusion of the C2–C7 vertebrae. All these procedures were performed in other hospitals, and no previous anaesthetic records were available.

Clinical examination

An airway examination showed:

- Fixed flexion of the cervical spine.
- An inter-incisor gap of 3cm.

- Mallampati score was 3.
- She weighed 60kg and her body mass index (BMI) was 22kg/m².

Investigations

- ECG — ventricular paced rhythm.
- Echocardiogram — severe mitral stenosis.
- Clotting studies showed a von Willebrand factor level of 70 international units/dL (range 50–200 international units/dL).

How this case was managed

Airway management

Because of the fixed cervical spine, the anaesthetist decided to secure the airway by performing awake fibreoptic intubation. The procedure was uneventful. Following the surgery, the patient was transferred to the cardiothoracic intensive care unit, intubated and ventilated. In the following days, the respiratory support was gradually weaned off. On the fourth postoperative day, the patient was considered ready for tracheal extubation.

Tracheal extubation

An anaesthetic consultant with expertise in the management of difficult airways was asked for advice and assistance. They decided to use an airway exchange catheter (AEC) for extubation.

The patient was placed in a sitting position. An 11FG, 83cm long AEC (Cook Medical, Bloomington, USA) was inserted through the tracheal tube. The tube was removed, and the AEC was left in the trachea and secured to the side of the face with tape (Figure 14.1). It was ensured that the tip of the catheter was 4cm above the carina. The catheter was well tolerated by the patient, maintaining good ventilation and oxygenation in the first 10 minutes. With time, it was noted that the patient's respiration was gradually becoming less efficient. Hypoventilation was confirmed by an increase in $PaCO_2$ in the arterial blood sample.

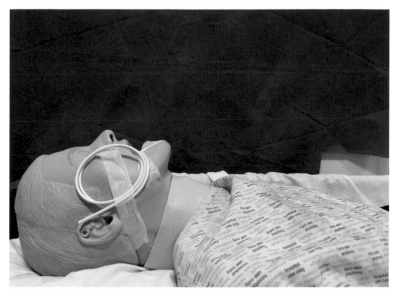

Figure 14.1. Cook® Airway Exchange Catheter™ secured to the face.

Approximately 45 minutes after the trachea was extubated, the patient's condition started to deteriorate rapidly. A decision to reintubate the trachea was made, and the consultant anaesthetist was called back to the intensive care unit to assist.

Following intravenous induction of general anaesthesia, suxamethonium was administered. A size 6mm ID tracheal tube was 'railroaded' over the AEC. Unexpectedly, obstruction to the passage of the tube was encountered. Repeated attempts of tube rotation failed to advance the tube but resulted in oesophageal intubation. Forceful advancement of the tube despite resistance may push the mid-segment of the catheter into the oesophagus (Figure 14.2). At this stage, the patient started desaturating to below 90%.

After the tube was removed the anaesthetist discovered that the obstruction was caused by a piece of adhesive tape previously used to secure the AEC (Figure 14.3), which had not been removed completely and was now stuck to the catheter.

A

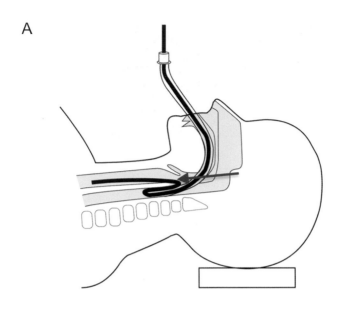

B

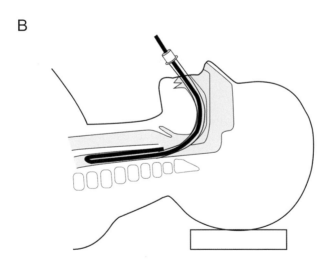

Figure 14.2. Oesophageal intubation over a catheter due to forceful advancement of the tracheal tube. A) Catheter looped around the posterior commissure (arrow). B) Catheter migrated to the oesophagus.

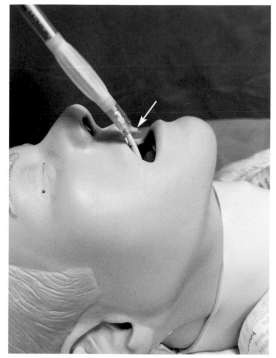

Figure 14.3. Piece of adhesive tape obstructing the passage of the tube over the catheter.

What was the next step?

Face mask ventilation using a self-inflating bag connected to 15L/minute of oxygen flow was commenced. A dose of non-depolarising muscle relaxant was administered to facilitate lung ventilation and further management of the airway.

Subsequently, two attempts were made at intubating the trachea using a King Vision™ channelled videolaryngoscope (Ambu, Copenhagen, Denmark; Figure 14.4). However, this failed to provide any view of the glottis. Bleeding into the airway was noted at this point. Oxygen saturations were successfully maintained with bag valve mask ventilation, which was still possible.

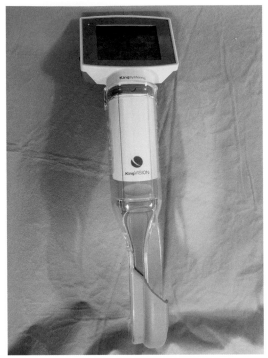

Figure 14.4. King Vision™ channelled videolaryngoscope.

A head and neck surgeon was called for assistance. With the patient's neck in a flexed position, it was extremely challenging for the head and neck consultant surgeon to perform the tracheostomy. With great difficulty, a size 7mm internal diameter tracheostomy tube was inserted. Ventilation through this tracheostomy tube resulted in surgical emphysema of the neck. It was realised that a false passage was created. Therefore, help was summoned from a second head and neck surgeon. At this stage, face mask ventilation became difficult due to the swelling of the submandibular region. A stab incision on the trachea was performed, and a bougie was inserted, allowing a 6mm standard tracheal tube to be 'railroaded' into position. The patient was then transferred to an operating theatre and a surgical tracheostomy was performed.

How would you manage this case differently?

- A plan for tracheal extubation is an essential part of airway management. Whenever the tracheal extubation is delayed and the patient is transferred to the intensive care unit after the operation, this plan should be clearly documented in the patient's notes and handed over to the intensive care staff. This can be planned using the Difficult Airway Society extubation algorithm, as referenced in Figure 20.3.
- If reintubation is necessary, optimum preparation for the procedure is vital. If it is performed on the intensive care unit, this includes special attention to factors such as the availability of difficult airway equipment, an assistant skilled in the use of that equipment and experienced in the management of failed intubation, positioning of the patient, adequate space and lighting, etc. This case demonstrates that minor technical issues can influence the patient's outcome.
- Difficult extubation should be planned during normal working hours when expert help is more likely to be available.
- The patient should be pre-oxygenated to extend the apnoeic window if problems with reintubation are encountered. This could be achieved using high-flow nasal oxygen.
- Front-of-neck access comprises Plan D of the Difficult Airway Society failed intubation algorithm (as shown in Figure 5.2) and should be implemented in a 'cannot intubate cannot oxygenate' situation.
- Front-of-neck access and even surgical tracheostomy may be extremely challenging in patients with abnormal anatomy of the neck due to cervical spine fixation, cervical spine disease causing a fixed neck flexion deformity, previous neck surgery, radiotherapy of the neck and a mass in the neck region. A front-of-neck access option may not be available in some patients.

Airway exchange catheter

Airway exchange catheters provide a safe method of reintubation in a patient with a potentially difficult airway. They are long, hollow, semi-rigid catheters with a small internal diameter that can be used for oxygen insufflation. There are many different types of airway exchange catheters commercially available, the most common of which are:

- Airway Exchange Catheter™ (Cook Critical Care, Bloomington, IN).
- Endotracheal Ventilation Catheter® (CardioMed, Gormley, Ontario, Canada).
- Tracheal Tube Exchanger™ (Sheridan Catheter Corporation, Argyle, NY).

Two airway exchange catheters (Figure 14.5) commonly used for reintubation are:

- 11Fr size with 83cm length. It has an internal diameter of 2.3mm and an external diameter of 3.7mm. Therefore, it allows 'railroading' of a tube of more than 4mm internal diameter.

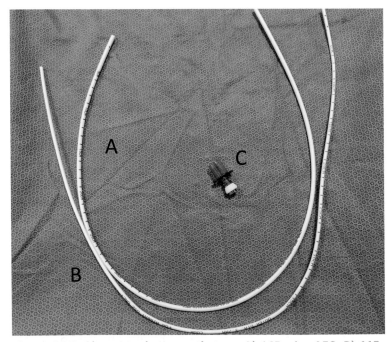

Figure 14.5. Airway exchange catheters. A) 14Fr size AEC. B) 11Fr size AEC. C) Rapi-Fit® connector.

- 14Fr size with 83cm length. It has an internal diameter of 3.7mm and external diameter of 4.7mm. Therefore, it allows 'railroading' of a tracheal tube of more than 5mm internal diameter. In adults, a tracheal tube of 5–6mm would be ideal for reintubation over these catheters. The larger the size of tube, tube impingement at the arytenoids is more likely.

A step-by-step method for inserting an airway exchange catheter is described below:

- Measure the depth (from the mid trachea to the lips or nose) of the AEC that needs to be inserted. The distal tip should lie above the carina. In adults, this should be no more than 25cm.
- At the point of extubation, insert a lubricated AEC into the endotracheal tube.
- Perform laryngoscopy and suction under direct vision and remove the endotracheal tube over the AEC.
- Use the breathing circuit connected to the 15mm Rapi-Fit® connector to confirm a leak around the AEC.
- Secure and clearly label the AEC.
- The patient should be nursed in a high dependency or critical care environment and remain nil by mouth until the AEC is removed. They may require supplemental oxygen via a face mask or nasal cannulae.
- A high flow of oxygen delivered through an AEC can cause barotrauma. Therefore, oxygen should be delivered through a face mask or nasal cannulae.
- AEC depth should be clearly documented in the patient records to assess for any displacement.
- If the patient is coughing, recheck the position of the catheter tip in relation to the carina. Lidocaine may be injected down the AEC to improve patient tolerance.
- The AEC should be removed when the airway is no longer at risk.

As with any piece of equipment, there are potential complications from the use of airway exchange catheters. These are often due to malposition/displacement of the catheter, barotrauma due to the use of a high flow of oxygen or the use of jet insufflation to provide oxygenation.

Occasionally, 'railroading' of the tracheal tube over the AEC may fail, and oesophageal intubation may still occur.

Front-of-neck access (FONA)

This procedure uses a simple scalpel, bougie, and tube technique to gain access to the trachea, allowing ventilation. The previously used needle cricothyroidotomy method is now not recommended due to multiple failed attempts to establish access and complications due to the technique. The equipment required for front-of-neck access includes:

- Size 10 scalpel (A).
- Bougie (B).
- Size 6mm endotracheal tube (C).

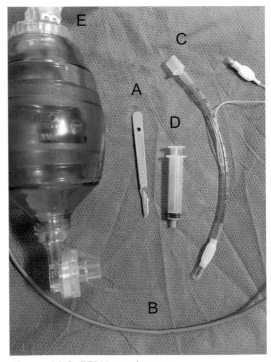

Figure 14.6. FONA equipment.

- Syringe (D).
- Self-inflating bag (E) connected to an oxygen source or breathing circuit.

These are depicted in Figure 14.6.

Figure 14.7 shows a flowchart of performing emergency front-of-neck access in a stepwise manner.

If, due to the patient's body habitus, the cricothyroid membrane cannot be identified on palpation, an initial vertical incision is made along the anterior surface of the neck from the sternal notch to the chin approximately 8–10cm long. Following this, the soft tissue is dissected using fingers until the anatomy is palpated. Once the anatomy is palpated, the steps are the same as shown in the flowchart (Figures 14.7-14.11).

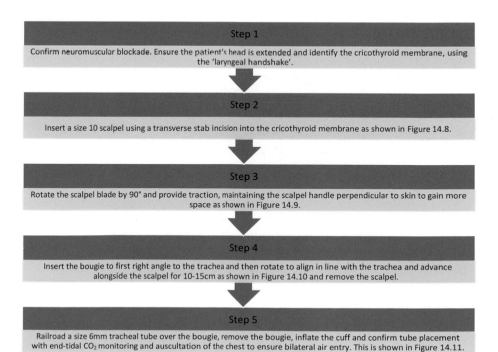

Step 1

Confirm neuromuscular blockade. Ensure the patient's head is extended and identify the cricothyroid membrane, using the 'laryngeal handshake'.

Step 2

Insert a size 10 scalpel using a transverse stab incision into the cricothyroid membrane as shown in Figure 14.8.

Step 3

Rotate the scalpel blade by 90° and provide traction, maintaining the scalpel handle perpendicular to skin to gain more space as shown in Figure 14.9.

Step 4

Insert the bougie to first right angle to the trachea and then rotate to align in line with the trachea and advance alongside the scalpel for 10-15cm as shown in Figure 14.10 and remove the scalpel.

Step 5

Railroad a size 6mm tracheal tube over the bougie, remove the bougie, inflate the cuff and confirm tube placement with end-tidal CO_2 monitoring and auscultation of the chest to ensure bilateral air entry. This is shown in Figure 14.11.

Figure 14.7. FONA flowchart.

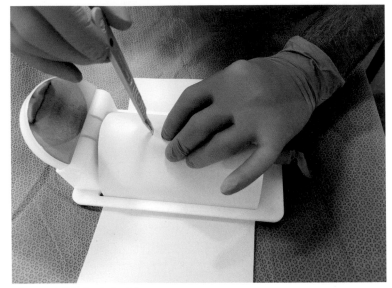

Figure 14.8. Stab incision.

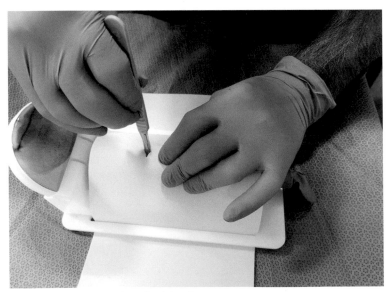

Figure 14.9. Rotated scalpel *in situ*.

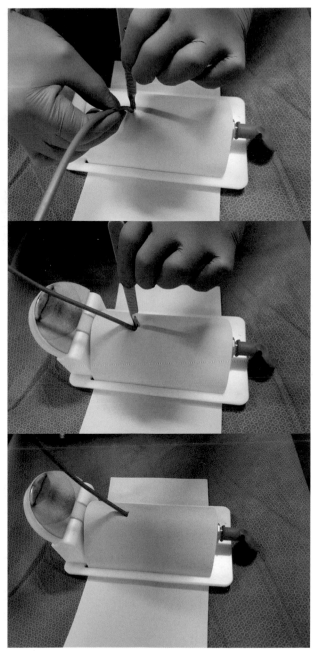

Figure 14.10. Bougie insertion.

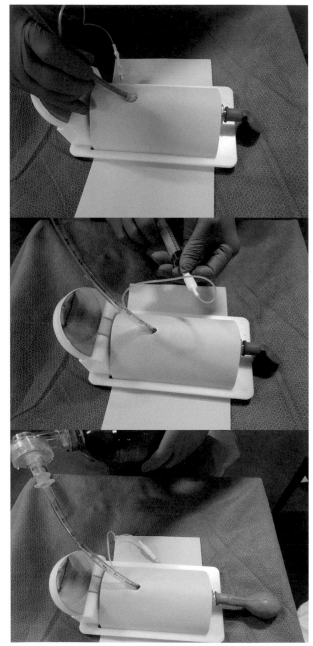

Figure 14.11. Tracheal tube 'railroaded' over the bougie.

What potential difficulties may be encountered while performing front-of-neck access?

- Excessive lateral traction leads to obstruction.
- The tip of the scalpel may slip out of the trachea when applying lateral traction.
- If the scalpel is not held perpendicularly to make the stab incision, there may be impingement against the side wall of the trachea or damage to local structures.
- Inserting the bougie vertically, not horizontally, may cause tracheal damage.
- The bougie may be inserted too deeply, leading to damage to the carina or leading to endobronchial intubation.

Key points

- The importance of planning for failure in cases of a known difficult airway cannot be overemphasised. This includes an extubation plan that should be documented if delayed and a reintubation plan.
- The possibility and ease of achieving front-of-neck access should be considered in all patients with a known difficult airway.
- Other forms of emergency tracheal access should be planned for and considered: front-of-neck access, surgical or percutaneous tracheostomy insertions.

References

1. Difficult Airway Society. CICO action cards. Available from: https://drive.google.com/file/d/1BKP6LlAMdu9_X4e9RiAGnw3JHuGJki6v/view.
2. Difficult Airway Society. Front of neck access – training video. Available from: https://das.uk.com/content/video/fona.
3. Royal College of Anaesthetists and Difficult Airway Society. 4th National Audit Project; March 2011. Available from: https://www.nationalauditprojects.org.uk/NAP4-Report.

Case scenario 15

Introduction

A 51-year-old male patient who had known hypopharyngeal cancer was awaiting a percutaneous endoscopic gastrostomy (PEG) feeding tube insertion. After returning to the ward from smoking, he was noted to develop stridor with concurrent desaturation.

He was urgently reviewed by an anaesthetic registrar, who promptly gave adrenaline and salbutamol nebulisers. The stridor subsequently improved with these measures; a decision was then taken to transfer the patient to the operating theatre for an emergency tracheostomy.

Past medical history

A quick review of electronic medical records revealed that he had a CT scan performed 3 months ago (Figure 15.1). He had initially presented to the head and neck clinic 10 months ago with a 'neck lump'. However, he failed to attend further appointments until 2 months ago when he presented to the emergency department after a collapse at work. He had a history of significant weight loss. History included smoking, alcohol, cocaine and cannabis use for more than 10 years. Recently he was dysphagic to both solids and fluids. Therefore, he was admitted for PEG feeding tube insertion.

Clinical examination

He had a red and tender neck lump on the right side measuring 3cm × 5cm.

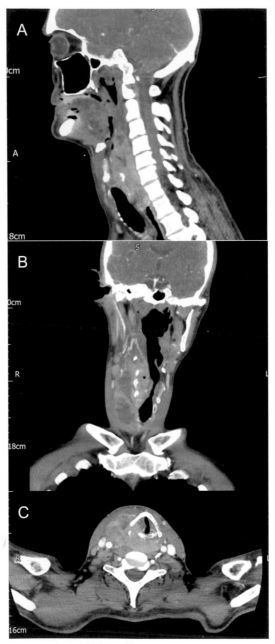

Figure 15.1. CT scan showing a large mass on the right side. A) Sagittal plane. B) Coronal plane. C) Transverse (axial) plane.

Investigations

A contrast CT scan showed a large heterogeneous mass lesion on the right side of the larynx. The lesion extended from the right lobe of the thyroid to the right side of the pharynx with expansion to the right parapharyngeal tissues. The airway deviated to the left with significant narrowing at the level of the larynx. The mass extended into the airway at the level of the cricoid cartilage. There was associated destruction of the cricoid and inferior thyroid cartilage on the right side.

How this case was managed

The anaesthetic registrar summoned help from a consultant anaesthetist. The key questions were:

- How would you secure their airway?
- Would you use an awake or asleep technique?
- How would you maintain oxygenation?
- What would you do if the initial plan failed?

The patient was transferred to the operating theatre with an anaesthetic escort. To assist with oxygenation, high-flow nasal oxygen was commenced. Following discussion with the multidisciplinary team, including the ENT surgeons and anaesthetic consultant, a plan was made to perform awake tracheal intubation as 'Plan A' with the ENT surgeon 'scrubbed' and ready to perform awake tracheostomy as 'Plan B'.

As part of the Plan A attempt, the airway was topicalised with 4% lidocaine spray. Sedation was given via a remifentanil target-controlled infusion (TCI) at 1–2ng/ml and a propofol TCI at 0.4–0.6µg/ml, titrated to maintain verbal contact with the patient. Awake intubation was attempted via the nasal route; however, it was difficult to advance the scope through the glottis. There was a large supraglottic mass that made it difficult to manoeuvre the tip of the scope. The glottic opening was narrow and, therefore, it was decided to abandon the awake intubation attempt. Therefore, Plan B 'awake tracheostomy' was activated.

The patient was positioned in full neck extension to allow surgical access. The surgeon infiltrated local anaesthetic into the surgical site. During these steps, the patient progressed from partial obstruction to complete obstruction with oxygenation saturation of 90% and started to desaturate.

As the patient had progressed to complete airway obstruction, the decision was made to perform an emergency front-of-neck (eFONA) procedure (Figure 14.7). A stab incision was made over the cricothyroid membrane, the bougie was inserted via the stab incision and a size 6mm cuffed tracheal tube was 'railroaded' over the bougie. The cuff was inflated and correct placement in the trachea was confirmed with a capnography trace. Once in place, the TCI dose of propofol and remifentanil was increased to induce general anaesthesia. Neuromuscular blockade was achieved with rocuronium, and the surgical team completed the tracheostomy.

The patient was transferred to the ITU when they were cautiously woken from sedation. The patient was discharged to the ward later that day and subsequently made a full recovery.

How would you manage this case differently?

- Awake tracheal intubation is a key skill for anaesthetists in the management of a predicted difficult airway. The 4th National Audit Project, jointly led by the Royal College of Anaesthetists and the Difficult Airway Society, showed that it is often under-utilised when there were clear indications to do so. The reasons for this are multifactorial.
- In the case described within this chapter, a difficult airway was recognised and awake tracheal intubation was selected as the primary airway strategy. Unfortunately, difficulty was encountered and the procedure was abandoned. This scenario highlights the importance of having a strategy before embarking on the procedure and having an alternative should difficulty be encountered. Indeed, the use of an algorithm or checklist is a well described tool for improving outcomes and performance in critical situations.
- The Difficult Airway Society has published guidelines on the management of awake tracheal intubation in adults that also

includes guidance on further management when the procedure is unsuccessful. Further details on awake tracheal intubation are described in case scenario 8. The main objective in this circumstance is to maintain oxygenation through any means possible, be it via a face mask, high-flow nasal oxygenation or a supraglottic airway device. A decision then needs to be made as to whether to postpone airway management or proceed if absolutely essential. If a decision is made to proceed, then the most appropriate option is most likely to be a front-of-neck access (FONA) using the most skilled operator, which would usually be a head and neck surgeon. The surgeon should be available and scrubbed before the initial ATI procedure takes place. If the circumstances and patient factors, e.g. anatomy, allow, then videolaryngoscopy may also be considered before a surgical airway.

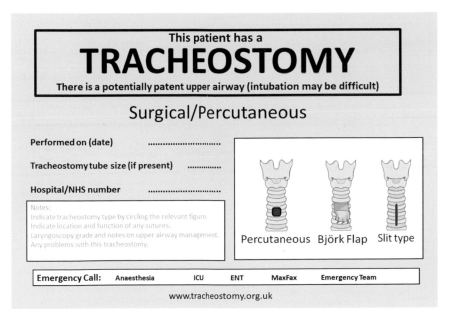

Figure 15.2. Bedhead tracheostomy poster and tracheostomy management algorithm. *Reproduced with permission from the National Tracheostomy Safety Project. Continued overleaf.*

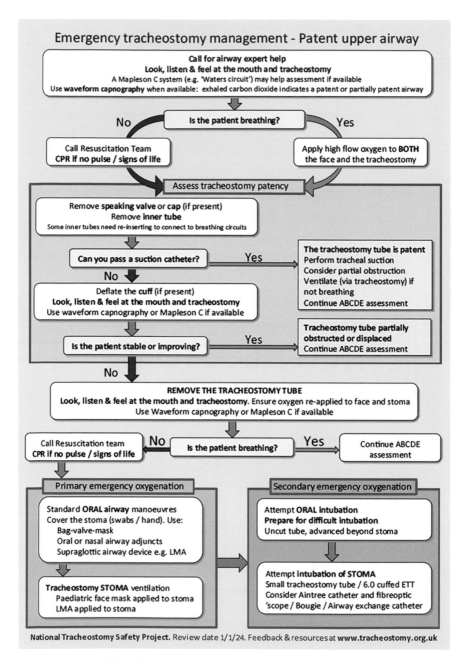

Figure 15.2. Bedhead tracheostomy poster and tracheostomy management algorithm. *Reproduced with permission from the National Tracheostomy Safety Project.*

- In the case described above, it would be useful to perform a nasendoscopy before the airway management attempt. This is often well tolerated with little or no topical anaesthesia and allows assessment of the upper airway anatomy and may highlight potential difficulties when trying to pass either the fibreoptic scope or the endotracheal tube. It is possible that the head and neck surgeons may have already performed a nasendoscopy and, if so, it is useful to see the images before airway management.

- A final but important element to consider is post-procedure management of the patient with a tracheostomy. It is crucial that this patient is cared for in an environment where both medical and nursing staff are experienced in tracheostomy management. This will always include the intensive care unit but, depending on local services, will include a head and neck/ENT ward.

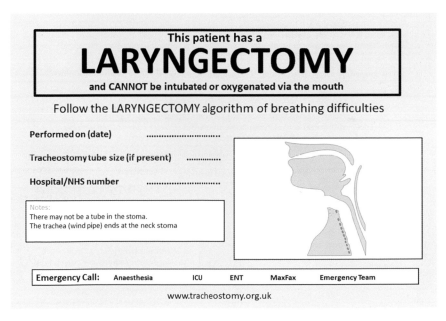

Figure 15.3. Bedhead laryngectomy poster and laryngectomy management algorithm. *Reproduced with permission from the National Tracheostomy Safety Project. Continued overleaf.*

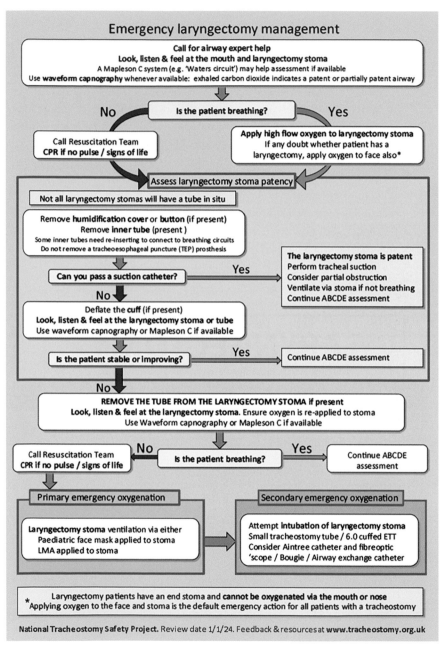

Figure 15.3. Bedhead laryngectomy poster and laryngectomy management algorithm. *Reproduced with permission from the National Tracheostomy Safety Project.*

- The National Tracheostomy Safety Project (NTSP) is a UK-based charity dedicated to improving standards around tracheostomy care and reducing clinical incidents. The NTSP provides a series of educational resources to aid the training of clinicians in tracheostomy management. There are also a series of 'bedhead' posters that describe the emergency management and contacts for an airway emergency in a patient with a tracheostomy. These posters are colour coded to rapidly identify if the patient has a patent upper airway and the appropriate management. These posters are shown in Figures 15.2 and 15.3.

Key points

- Awake tracheal intubation can fail. Therefore, a plan must be in place to manage failed awake tracheal intubation.
- Difficult Airway Society guidelines in managing awake tracheal intubation provide guidance in managing complications during awake tracheal intubation.
- Always be prepared for failure.
- Always mark the front-of-neck anatomy and site.

References

1. Ahmad I, El-Boghdadly K, Bhagrath R, et al. Difficult Airway Society guidelines for awake tracheal intubation (ATI) in adults. Anaesthesia 2020; 75(4): 509-28.

2. Cook TM, Woodall N, Frerk C; 4th National Audit Project. Major complications of airway management in the UK: results of the 4th National Audit Project of the Royal College of Anaesthetists and the Difficult Airway Society. Part 1: anaesthesia. Br J Anaesth 2011; 106(5): 617-31.

3. Jones CPL, Fawker-Corbett J, Groom P, et al. Human factors in preventing complications in anaesthesia: a systematic review. Anaesthesia 2018; 73(suppl 1): 12-24.

4. Leslie D, Stacey M. Awake intubation. Contin Educ Anaesth Crit Care Pain 2015; 15(2): 64-7.

At the end of the surgery, the patient was turned into the supine position and anaesthesia was discontinued. The patient was slow to wake up from the anaesthetic, and it was approximately 30 minutes before spontaneous breathing was noted.

The breathing pattern was noticed to be abnormal, with 'jerky' movements and a low tidal volume. To rule out the incomplete reversal of neuromuscular blockade, sugammadex was given at the appropriate dose. The situation failed to improve, with the end-tidal carbon dioxide rising to 10kPa.

How this situation was managed

Given the history of asthma, a presumed diagnosis of acute bronchospasm was made. Anaesthesia was reinduced with intravenous propofol and neuromuscular blockade using rocuronium. Anaesthesia was maintained with a sevoflurane inhalation agent.

Despite these measures, the patient remained difficult to ventilate with tidal volumes of no more than 200ml achieved and high peak airway pressure persisted.

What are the possible causes?

- Partial occlusion of the breathing circuit.
- Obstruction of the tracheal tube.
- Bronchospasm.
- Anaphylaxis.
- Pneumothorax.
- Pulmonary oedema.
- Endobronchial intubation or migration of the endotracheal tube.

Further anaesthetic support was summoned, and further bronchospasm management was given in the form of endotracheal salbutamol, intravenous adrenaline and intravenous magnesium. There was minimal improvement following these interventions.

The heat and moisture exchange (HME) filter was noticed to be wet and was changed. At this point, the tidal volumes recovered to the normal expected for the patient's weight. Peak pressures also returned to normal.

The patient was ventilated for a further 30 minutes to normalise the high carbon dioxide. The second dose of neuromuscular blockade was reversed with sugammadex, and then the patient was extubated.

A further monitoring period in the theatre for 30 minutes was undertaken to ensure stability, and then he was transferred to recovery.

This issue had not been recognised or suspected earlier as there was no increase in airway pressure or difficulty in ventilation until spontaneous ventilation had begun.

How would you manage this case differently?

Clinical aspects

- There are several possible differential diagnoses in this case; therefore, it is important to follow a structured approach in what will rapidly become a high-stress environment. In this case, the primary problem was that of high airway pressure.
- High airway pressure can be due to a cause outside the patient or due to a problem outside of the airway device to the anaesthetic machine. Important causes include airway obstruction (secretions, mucous plug or blood clot), obstruction in the breathing system, malfunction of a ventilator, AL valves or anaesthetic machine. A systematic approach (Figure 16.1) for investigating the cause of high airway pressure will allow earlier identification of the problem. The authors would recommend the use of the Quick Reference Handbook (QRH) — published by the Association of Anaesthetists — Section 2-3, on the management of increased airway pressure.
- In this case, the problem was within the anaesthetic circuit, specifically the HME filter. Following a protocol such as that found in the Quick Reference Handbook would identify this rapidly, especially

- Increase fresh gas flow and give 100% oxygen
- Rapidly check the breathing system
- Hand ventilate, confirm the feel of the bag and check inspired/expired tidal volume

Ventilation improves; the problem should be in the breathing system or machine

AIRWAY

- Check airway for obstruction (pass a suction catheter), kinking of tube, listen for noise, leak
- Check capnography
- Ventilate lungs using a self-inflating bag connected directly to the airway device. If the ventilation improves, the problem should be with the catheter mount, filter or breathing system, ventilator or the machine

BREATHING

- Look for bilateral chest movement, auscultate for breath sounds, check airway pressure, SPO2, inspired/expired tidal volume/airway pressure
- Check depth of anaesthesia and neuromuscular blockade

CIRCULATION

- Check HR, rhythm, BP and peripheral perfusion

Problem persisting

Call for expert help, arrange for a chest X-ray, 12-lead ECG, chest ultrasound

Figure 16.1. A systematic approach at investigating the cause for high airway pressure.

if the endotracheal tube is connected directly to a separate anaesthetic circuit such as a Mapleson C or a self-filling bag (isolating the anaesthetic machine and breathing system). If the problem resolves, important patient-related causes, such as pneumothorax, bronchospasm, and inadequate depth of anaesthesia, can be excluded. In this case, it may have prevented reinducing anaesthesia or neuromuscular blockade from being readministered.

- There are several case reports of the HME filter becoming blocked by secretions or a defect within the device itself. During the height of the COVID-19 pandemic, blockage of the HME filters within the ventilator circuit was a particular issue leading to a patient safety alert being issued by NHS England.
- Partial blockage of the filter can increase resistance to gas flow and prevent adequate gas exchange. Identification of the HME filter as the cause can be difficult as it is often hidden under drapes and, even on close inspection, it may be difficult to see that it is clogged with secretions or other debris. To prevent this, the filter should be placed higher than the patient's lungs, with the filter layer orientated vertically rather than horizontally.
- One of the main issues encountered was that of poor tidal volume at emergence from anaesthesia. There are many possible causes for this, and airway or anaesthetic circuit obstruction has been discussed above. Other causes to consider include inadequate reversal of neuromuscular blockade, opiate-induced respiratory depression, hypothermia and effects from either thoracic or abdominal surgery.

Human factors

- An important aspect of this case was the prolonged nature of the surgery. This leads to a high risk of fatigue among all members of staff involved in the patient's care. From an anaesthetic point of view, this is a prolonged period of mental alertness required to monitor the patient. Fatigue has a negative impact on the performance of an individual and a team, substantially increasing the risk of errors occurring within clinical practice.

- In this case, the emergency occurred at the end of a prolonged procedure when the performance of the team or any individual would not have been at its peak. The element of diagnostic overshadowing when asthma was treated rather than identifying the true cause may bear some relationship to the fatigue probably being experienced.
- A full discussion of human factors and fatigue within anaesthesia is beyond the scope of this book. It is important to try and be aware of fatigue when possible, take breaks and build a culture in which help can be easily accessed. Issues on human factors in emergency airway management are discussed in Case scenario 22.

Key points

- Consider a wide range of differentials when managing airway emergencies, and be aware of diagnostic overshadowing.
- In this case, the presence of asthma in the past medical history led to the exclusion of all other differentials and fixation on bronchospasm.
- Issues may occur with the equipment rather than with the patient.
- It is important to use a systematic approach in evaluating the cause of high airway pressure at emergence.
- It's important to change the HME filter after a long case; this is especially the case following prone positioning, as secretions tend to pool in the endotracheal tube and block the HME filter.

References

1. Association of Anaesthetists. Increased airway pressure. Quick Reference Handbook 2019. Available from: https://anaesthetists.org/Home/Resources-publications/Safety-alerts/Anaesthesia-emergencies/Quick-Reference-Handbook.

2.   Kelly FE, Frerk C, Bailey CR, *et al.* Implementing human factors in anaesthesia: guidance for clinicians, departments and hospitals: guidelines from the Difficult Airway Society and the Association of Anaesthetists. *Anaesthesia* 2023; 78(4): 458-78.

3.   Kelly FE, Frerk C, Bailey CR, *et al.* Human factors in anaesthesia: a narrative review. *Anaesthesia* 2023; 78(4): 479-90.

4.   Lawes EG. Hidden hazards and dangers associated with the use of HME/filters in breathing circuits. Their effect on toxic metabolite production, pulse oximetry and airway resistance. *Br J Anaesth* 2003; 91(2): 249-64.

5.   Wilkes AR. Heat and moisture exchangers and breathing system filters: their use in anaesthesia and intensive care. Part 2 - practical use, including problems, and their use with paediatric patients. *Anaesthesia* 2011; 66(1): 40-51.

Case scenario 17

Introduction

A 26-year-old motorcyclist was admitted to the accident and emergency department after a collision with a car. On the scene, he was found with a helmet strap pulled up around the neck.

On admission to the hospital, the patient was conscious. His main presenting complaints were upper back pain and severe breathing difficulties.

Past medical history

He had no other past medical history to note.

Clinical examination

He was able to talk, although in a hoarse voice, and was complaining of breathing difficulties. There was no blood or secretions in the oral cavity or the oropharynx.

His vital signs were:

- Respiratory rate was 20 breaths/minute.
- The pulse rate was 108 beats/minute.
- Blood pressure was 115/76mmHg.
- The pulse oximetry waveform trace was poor quality, so 15L/minute of oxygen was administered through a non-rebreathe mask.

Chest auscultation was normal. The patient remained tachycardic but haemodynamically stable.

Investigations

- His arterial blood gas sample showed a PaO_2 of 39.1kPa and a $PaCO_2$ of 5.6kPa on a 15L non-rebreathe mask.
- A trauma CT revealed a burst fracture of the T3 vertebral body with depression of the superior end plate, a compression fracture of the T4 and T5 vertebral bodies, with a prevertebral haematoma. There was also a very small pneumothorax, several mild lung contusions and a suspected single rib fracture. Some local oedema around the larynx was also reported.

How this case was managed

Despite adequate analgesia, the patient continued to complain of considerable difficulties in breathing. There was no stridor and the breathing pattern appeared normal, but the patient's voice was hoarse. An ENT review was, therefore, requested.

The ENT surgeon reviewed the CT scan together with the radiology consultant. This joint review resulted in a suspicion that the dyspnoea may be caused by a large prevertebral haematoma of the superior, middle and posterior mediastinum compressing the bilateral recurrent laryngeal nerves.

The patient was transferred to the operating theatre, where a flexible nasendoscopy was performed. The procedure was well tolerated by the patient. It revealed a large haematoma above the right vocal cord and bilateral vocal cord paresis, with vocal cords in the paramedian position.

A tracheostomy was performed by the ENT surgeon under local anaesthesia. After the procedure, the patient was transferred to the high dependency unit. He required no respiratory support and was discharged to the ward 24 hours later.

How would you manage this case differently?

- Documentation of injuries sustained by the patient could use recognised classification systems, such as the Schaefer and Fuhrman classification in this case (shown in Table 17.1). This may give more information to develop an airway strategy.

Table 17.1. Schaefer and Fuhrman classification of severity of laryngeal injury.	
Class	**Severity of injury**
Class 0	Normal larynx.
Class 1	Minor endolaryngeal haematoma or lacerations without detectable fractures, no airway compromise.
Class 2	More severe oedema, haematoma, minor mucosal disruption without exposed cartilage, or non-displaced fractures. Varying degrees of airway compromise.
Class 3	Massive oedema, large mucosal lacerations, exposed cartilage, displaced fractures or vocal cord immobility. Airway compromise.
Class 4	Same as group 3, but more severe, with disruption of the anterior larynx, unstable fractures, two or more fracture lines, or severe mucosal injuries. Requires the use of a mould for stabilisation.
Class 5	Complete laryngotracheal separation.

- Consider co-administration of intravenous dexamethasone/ nebulised adrenaline to reduce any further oedema.

- Making a clear plan for tracheostomy management — plans for emergency management and decannulation plans if emergency management of a tracheostomy is required.
- In a patient who is not cooperative, agitated and has a reduced Glasgow Coma Scale (GCS), local anaesthesia may not be tolerated and general anaesthesia may be required. A good airway management strategy and preparation are essential.

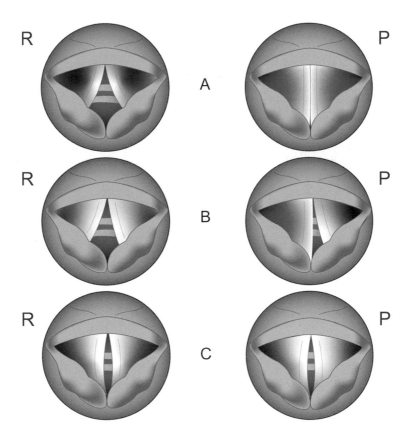

Figure 17.1. Vocal cord positions during respiration (R) and during phonation (P) based on laryngeal nerve injury. A) Normal. B) Unilateral vocal cord paralysis (paralysed cord in the paramedian position). C) Bilateral vocal cord paralysis.

The position of the vocal cords either on radiology or on clinical examination, in this case fine nasendoscopy, may give an indication of the level of the lesion. The different variations of vocal cord position are illustrated in Figure 17.1.

Another way to identify the nerve affected can be to use signs and symptoms exhibited by the patient. Unilateral and bilateral lesions can be identified, allowing the development of a complete airway management plan for these patients. The signs and symptoms for each nerve supplying the vocal cords are explained in Table 17.2 below.

Table 17.2. Laryngeal nerve injuries and their effects.

Nerve injury	Signs and symptoms
Vagus nerve (involves both the superior laryngeal nerve and recurrent laryngeal nerve)	Unilateral: hoarseness Bilateral: aphonia
Recurrent laryngeal nerve (chronic): aphonia	Unilateral: hoarseness, change in voice Bilateral (acute): stridor, respiratory distress, complete airway obstruction
Superior laryngeal nerve	Unilateral: minimal effects Bilateral: hoarseness, tiring of voice

Key points

- Recurrent laryngeal nerve palsy is a rare cause of dyspnoea. It is even more unusual in an acute trauma scenario. The case is a good illustration of the fact that the presence of one pathology does not exclude other problems.
- A flexible nasendoscopy is a simple procedure that is well tolerated by patients. The skill is relatively easy to learn and is a useful tool that aids the assessment of the airway and decision making.

References

1.   Fuhrman GM, Stieg FH, III, Buerk CA. Blunt laryngeal trauma: classification and management protocol. *J Trauma* 1990; 30(1): 87-92.

2.   Latoo M, Lateef M, Nawaz I, Ali I. Bilateral recurrent laryngeal nerve palsy following blunt neck trauma. *Indian J Otolaryngol Head Neck Surg* 2007; 59(3): 298-99.

3.   Moonsamy P, Sachdeva UM, Morse CR. Management of laryngotracheal trauma. *Ann Cardiothorac Surg* 2018; 7(2): 210-6.

4..   Sanapala A, Nagaraju M, Rao LN, Nalluri K. Management of bilateral recurrent laryngeal nerve paresis after thyroidectomy. *Anesth Essays Res* 2015; 9(2): 251-3.

5.   Schaefer SD. The acute management of external laryngeal trauma. A 27-year experience. *Arch Otolaryngol Head Neck Surg* 1992; 118(6): 598-604.

Case scenario 18

Introduction

A 70-year-old woman underwent a hemi-glossectomy, neck dissection and reconstruction with a forearm radial free flap 12 days ago. A tracheostomy was performed at the time of surgery. Her postoperative course was stormy, requiring a return to the theatre for a tongue debridement 24 hours ago.

The patient was placed in the head and neck ward, initially on room air, breathing spontaneously via the stoma with a tracheostomy *in situ*. For the last 2 hours, the ward staff have noticed profuse bleeding from the tracheostomy site.

The head and neck surgical team were called urgently to review the patient. While awaiting surgical review, the ward team increased the oxygen to 15L via the tracheostomy mask.

Past history

She had no other past medical history to note.

Clinical examination

- Heart rate (HR): 98 bpm, blood pressure (BP): 110/76mmHg.
- Respiratory rate 24 bpm, partially obstructed breathing.
- Peripheral oxygen saturation 94% on 15L/minute oxygen via a tracheostomy mask.
- Mouth opening 25mm.

To tamponade the bleeding site, the tracheostomy tube cuff was inflated. On review, the surgical team decided to explore the tracheostomy site to secure the haemostasis. The surgical plan required the removal of the

149

tracheostomy tube to explore the bleeding site and secure the trachea intubation via the oral route.

Intravenous access was secured, and 1L of warm Hartmann's solution was administered. Blood was sent for a full blood count, clotting screen and crossmatch of 2 units of blood were requested.

Investigations

Postoperative routine investigations were within the normal range.

How this case was managed

The main anaesthetic concerns were:

- Airway bleeding.
- Altered airway anatomy from previous surgery.
- Ongoing haemorrhage.

A decision was made to induce general anaesthesia. Pre-oxygenation was performed via a Mapleson C circuit attached to the auxiliary oxygen outlet, connected directly to the tracheostomy; a mask connected to the anaesthetic circle system was applied to the patient's mouth.

General anaesthesia was induced using a balanced technique of fentanyl 100μg and propofol 100mg until loss of consciousness. Muscle relaxation was provided using 70mg rocuronium.

Due to concerns about altered anatomy, a C-MAC® videolaryngoscope with D-Blade was used. Oral lavage was performed guided by the videolaryngoscope. The laryngoscope blade could only be inserted into the left side of the oral cavity due to the previous right hemi-glossectomy.

The airway anatomy was difficult to visualise due to the pooling of secretions and blood in the pharynx. Once the C-MAC® D-Blade was inserted, there was not enough room to insert a Yankauer suction tube. A 12FG suction catheter was passed into the oral cavity to clear the secretions.

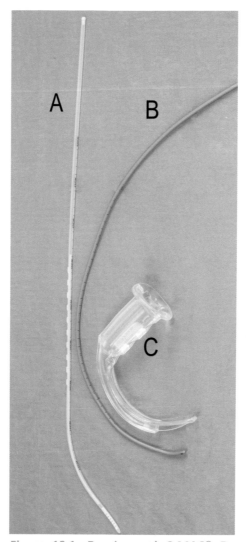

Figure 18.1. Bougies and C-MAC® D-Blade. A) Flexible Tip Bougie® has slider tabs that allow the tip to be flexed and retroflexed. B) Frova™ intubating catheter (bougie). C) C-MAC® D-Blade.

The overall concern was that deflation of the tracheostomy cuff would release the tamponade effect and precipitate uncontrolled bleeding. To maintain control of the airway, a Flexible Tip Bougie® (Figure 18.1) was placed above the tracheostomy tube cuff. A head and neck surgeon was scrubbed, ready to intervene if necessary.

When the Flexible Tip Bougie® was in place just above the cuff, the cuff was deflated, and the bougie advanced further beyond it. An endotracheal tube was loaded onto the bougie and then advanced into the trachea as the tracheostomy tube was removed.

Subsequent surgery to control the bleeding passed without further complications, and haemostasis was achieved. A tracheostomy tube was reinserted into the surgical stoma site at the end of the surgery. At that point, there was a sudden desaturation to 80%.

What was the next step?

It was confirmed that the patient was desaturating. The airway pressure alarm sounded with a peak airway pressure of 40cmH$_2$O. Ventilation was switched to a manual bag, which confirmed difficult ventilation. On auscultation, it was difficult to hear breath sounds.

Possible causes at this point:

- Blood clot from previous bleeding.
- Pneumothorax.
- Severe bronchospasm.
- Misplaced or blocked tracheostomy tube.

A rapid assessment was performed using the Quick Reference Handbook algorithm 'increased airway pressure'. In the context of airway bleeding, it was felt that obstruction from a blood clot or other foreign debris related to surgery was most likely. Bronchoscopy was carried out via the tracheostomy that showed an obstructing clot in the right main bronchus. Using cautious suction, this was removed which resolved the situation, with oxygen saturation subsequently improving and airway pressure returning to baseline.

How would you manage this case differently?

- This was a particularly challenging case, with an impending airway obstruction adding to the urgency of management. There are several approaches to the management of this case that will depend on the equipment and skill set of the operator.
- An alternative strategy would be to consider using a fibreoptic scope before intubation attempts. This would allow the airway anatomy and potential problems to be assessed. This requires a cooperative patient; however, a small scope is usually tolerated well via the nose.
- An awake technique to secure the airway could also be used. A fibreoptic scope could be used to pass an endotracheal tube via the oral or nasal route once sufficient topicalisation had been undertaken.
- A high-flow nasal oxygen delivery system could be used simultaneously, increasing the fraction of inspired oxygen, potentially prolonging the time available to secure the airway and aiding in the spread of the local anaesthetic topicalisation. This would have the advantage of preserving the patient's own respiratory effort while securing the airway. In this case, the scope could be positioned through the vocal cords up to the location of the tracheostomy tube. The tracheostomy tube could then be removed, and the preloaded endotracheal tube passed down the trachea beyond the stoma site.
- Another potential strategy would be to use the fibreoptic scope to assess for correct placement of the endotracheal tube. This could then be used after the tracheostomy tube insertion. This gives the operator reassurance that the endotracheal tube and tracheostomy tube are not malpositioned. For the tracheostomy, it would also allow bleeding or damage to the trachea to be assessed.

Tracheostomy bleeding

Bleeding from a tracheostomy, as in this case, is common. A UK NCEPOD report published in 2014 demonstrated major bleeding in 1.2% and minor bleeding in 4.4% of patients. Morbidity and mortality are increased in those with a tracheostomy if they have an episode of bleeding.

The causes of tracheostomy bleeding are often multifactorial but can be categorised into 'early' and 'late' bleeding based on when the stoma was formed. The following information is based on the National Tracheostomy Safety Project guidance.

Early bleeding:

- Originating from the skin.
- Related to the thyroid gland.
- Related to anticoagulant or antiplatelet therapy.

Late bleeding:

- Erosion into a large artery, often the innominate artery.
- Granulation tissue.
- Trauma from suction catheters.

All bleeding from a tracheostomy should be reviewed promptly by an experienced clinician. This should involve a member of the surgical team or intensive care team, depending on the context.

Recommended actions:

- Sit the patient up.
- Administer supplemental oxygen.
- Measure vital signs.
- If there are signs of active bleeding, call for help from the local emergency call/cardiac arrest team based on local policy.
- Notify the responsible surgical team (this should be documented on the tracheostomy bedhead sign).
- When there is major bleeding, signs of hypoxia or respiratory distress, activate emergency team-based local protocols.

When there are signs of a major arterial bleed, then hyperinflate the tracheostomy cuff or use direct digital compression of the bleeding point. Do not deflate a cuff that is inflated, as this may be providing a tamponade effect.

Any sign of airway compromise should prompt urgent intervention by those with advanced airway skills to secure the airway, with subsequent transfer to theatre for ongoing stabilisation and assessment. It is important to involve either ENT or maxillofacial surgeons to guide further management.

Key points

- Collaborative working with head and neck/ENT surgeons in forming an airway plan is imperative.
- A rapid and comprehensive assessment of the patient should be undertaken using the A–E approach and any abnormalities should be treated as they are found.
- Parallel resuscitation — in this case a shocked patient should be given blood while the initial assessment is continuing.
- Any bleeding of any volume from a tracheostomy site must be thoroughly evaluated and managed appropriately.

References

1. Association of Anaesthetists. Increased airway pressure. Quick Reference Handbook. 2019. Available from: https://anaesthetists.org/Home/Resources-publications/Safety-alerts/Anaesthesia-emergencies /Quick-Reference-Handbook.

2. Warrilow S, Ward J, McMurray K. Tracheostomy emergencies: bleeding; 2018. Available from: https://www.tracheostomy.org.uk/storage/files/Bleeding.pdf.

3. Wilkinson KA, Martin IC, Freeth H, et al. On the right trach? A review of the care received by patients who underwent a tracheostomy; 2014. Available from: https://www.ncepod.org.uk/2014report1/ downloads/OnTheRightTrach_Summary.pdf.

Atracurium was used due to the earlier administration of sugammadex. The reinforced tube was removed, and tracheal intubation was completed using a new 8mm internal diameter standard tracheal tube. On close inspection, the original tube was significantly deformed.

Following reintubation, the patient was extubated successfully. Supplemental oxygen was administered using a venturi mask at an $FiO_2 = 0.4$. Arterial blood gas is shown below in Box 19.1.

Box 19.1. Arterial blood gas results.

- pH   7.34
- PaO_2 15.6kPa
- $PaCO_2$ 5.2kPa
- SaO_2 99%
- Base excess (BE)   1.2mmol/L
- $HCO3^-$ 26mmol/L
- Lactate   1.2mmol/L

Given the risk of swelling due to multiple airway manipulations and the risk of negative pressure pulmonary oedema due to inspiration against the obstruction, it was decided to observe the patient in the critical care area for the next 12 hours. The next day the patient was deemed well enough to transfer to the ward.

How would you manage this case differently?

- This case had several differential diagnoses, and it is important to follow a structured approach in what will rapidly become a high-stress environment. In this case, the primary problem was that of high airway pressure (as discussed in Case scenario 16). For further details, refer to the Quick Reference Handbook of the Association of Anaesthetists, Section 2–3, on the management of increased airway pressure.

- Passing a suction catheter via the endotracheal tube identified the partial occlusion and prompted the removal of the damaged tube in favour of mask ventilation, supraglottic airway device or reintubation as appropriate. In this case, it is likely that using a pressure support mode when spontaneous effort had resumed and then manual ventilation provided sufficient pressure to partially overcome the partial obstruction within the tube, and so it improved the tidal volumes to an extent, compared with the patient's own respiratory effort against an obstruction.

- One differential for this scenario was an inadequate reversal of the neuromuscular blockade. The aminosteroid agent rocuronium had been used as the primary muscle relaxant. To reverse this, a dose of sugammadex had been given; a dose of 2mg/kg is recommended for routine reversal with an additional dose of 4mg/kg if inadequate reversal has been achieved guided by neuromuscular monitoring. For immediate reversal following intubation, the manufacturer recommends a dose of 16mg/kg. In this case, a further dose could have been given if the neuromuscular monitoring had shown no improvement and other causes had been excluded.

- The use of sugammadex is often effective for the reversal of neuromuscular blockade. However, it does present the anaesthetist with a potential problem if neuromuscular blockade needs to be re-established, as in this case. Sugammadex is cleared from the body at a rate proportional to the glomerular filtration rate, so there may be residual free sugammadex molecules present for some time. The consequence of this is either a delayed or complete failure of onset of neuromuscular blockade should an aminosteroid (rocuronium or vecuronium) agent be given. One option is to use a repeat dose of rocuronium, with doses of 0.6–1.2mg/kg being used. This gives the option of further reversal with sugammadex. Another option is the use of an agent from a different class. In this case, atracurium (a benzylisoquinolinium) was used. This avoids the interaction with sugammadex and the concern on dosing but does preclude rapid reversal should this become necessary.

- Given this patient's history of asthma, it is important to consider bronchospasm as a cause for the increased airway pressure encountered in this case. There was no wheeze present on auscultation (check main body); however, in the presence of poor tidal volumes, this may not be clinically apparent. The full management of bronchospasm during anaesthesia is covered in the Quick Reference Handbook.

Extubation planning

Extubation is a critical part of anaesthesia, and appropriate planning is necessary to minimise problems. The Difficult Airway Society has published a series of guidelines that help stratify and prepare for extubation. The following is based on their guidance.

In this case, consideration of a bite block may have prevented the partial occlusion of the tube (Figure 19.2). Several devices have been used for this purpose, including a Guedel airway or a rolled gauze. Related to this, the airway can be exchanged for a second-generation supraglottic airway device, for example an i-gel®, during deep anaesthesia. This has the advantage of providing airway support as well as providing a bite block upon emergence.

Awake or deep extubation is something that should be planned. Awake extubation has the advantage of the return of airway reflexes and tone. Deep extubation reduces the likelihood of coughing and the haemodynamic effects of extubation. This has the considerable downside of an increased risk of airway obstruction.

Pharmacological strategies are increasingly used to promote a smooth emergence from anaesthesia and subsequent extubation. The short-acting opiate remifentanil is commonly used for this purpose, but requires experience and careful titration. A target level of 2–4ng/ml is commonly used.

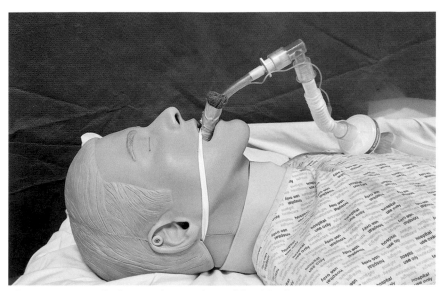

Figure 19.2. A rolled gauze inserted as a bite block.

Lidocaine has been used for this purpose previously. There are variable results, but there is some evidence to suggest that either intravenous lidocaine or lidocaine applied to the endotracheal cuff can reduce coughing upon extubation. There is debate whether topical lidocaine has these advantages.

One final agent to consider is dexmedetomidine. This is an alpha-2 adrenergic receptor antagonist that has sedative properties without respiratory depression. This is gaining increasing popularity in this context for achieving a smooth emergence and extubation following general anaesthesia with the added benefit of reducing coughing. Dexmedetomidine is also gaining favour within the intensive care environment as a way to support extubation in the context of delirium.

Key points

- Reinforced tracheal tubes have reinforced metal coils that make them less likely to become kinked. However, if the patient bites on the tube, the metal coils will be irreversibly deformed, causing airway obstruction.
- Consider the routine use of bite blocks for all extubations.
- Remifentanil running at 2–4ng/ml of effect site concentration (Ce) allows smooth extubation.
- Consideration of other techniques have also been proposed, such as dexmedetomidine intravenous or topical lidocaine; or lidocaine applied inside the tracheal tube cuff.

References

1. Association of Anaesthetists. Increased airway pressure. Quick Reference Handbook. 2019. Available from: https://anaesthetists.org/Home/Resources-publications/Safety-alerts/Anaesthesia-emergencies/Quick-Reference-Handbook.

2. Difficult Airway Society Extubation Guidelines Group, Popat M, Mitchell V, et al. Difficult Airway Society Guidelines for the management of tracheal extubation. Anaesthesia 2012; 67(3): 318-40.

3. Iwasaki H, Renew JR, Kunisawa T, Brull SJ. Preparing for the unexpected: special considerations and complications after sugammadex administration. BMC Anesthesiol 2017; 17(1): 140.

4. Siobal MS, Kallet RH, Kivett VA, Tang JF. Use of dexmedetomidine to facilitate extubation in surgical intensive-care-unit patients who failed previous weaning attempts following prolonged mechanical ventilation: a pilot study. Respir Care 2006; 51(5): 492-6.

5. Tung A, Fergusson NA, Ng N, et al. Medications to reduce emergence coughing after general anaesthesia with tracheal intubation: a systematic review and network meta-analysis. Br J Anaesth 2020; S0007-0912(20)30012-X.

6. Watkins J, Lee D, White WA Jr, Mundy S. Effects of topical lidocaine on successful extubation time among patients undergoing elective carotid endarterectomies. AANA J 2012; 80(2): 99-104.

7. Woods BD, Sladen RN. Perioperative considerations for the patient with asthma and bronchospasm. Br J Anaesth 2009; 103(suppl 1): i57-i65.

8. Yang SS, Wang NN, Postonogova T, et al. Intravenous lidocaine to prevent postoperative airway complications in adults: a systematic review and meta-analysis. Br J Anaesth 2020; 124(3): 314-23.

Case scenario 20

Introduction

A 52-year-old male patient presented to the emergency department following a road traffic collision. Following a trauma CT scan, the following injuries were identified:

- A fracture of an odontoid peg.
- An unstable fracture of the T6 vertebra.
- Fractures of the hip.
- Clavicle fracture.
- Bilateral rib fractures.

At 24 hours later, he was scheduled to undergo an open reduction and internal fixation of the clavicle, a split skin graft and a halo vest immobilisation of the cervical spine.

Past medical history

He had no other past medical history to note.

Clinical examination

Airway assessment revealed:

- Mallampati score of 2.
- Mouth opening of three finger breadths.
- Jaw protrusion was class A (able to protrude the bottom incisors beyond the upper incisors).

A further anaesthetic assessment revealed the patient was adequately starved. He weighed 70kg, with a BMI of 27kg/m^2. There were no symptoms of spinal cord compression.

Investigations

- Trauma CT imaging as described above.
- A full blood count and renal function were all within the normal range.

How this case was managed

General anaesthesia was induced using a modified rapid sequence induction technique with fentanyl, propofol and rocuronium. The neck collar was removed before the induction, and manual in-line stabilisation of the head was used.

Direct laryngoscopy with a size 4 Macintosh blade showed a Cormack and Lehane grade 2 view of the larynx. A reinforced endotracheal tube was easily passed into the trachea over a bougie. Anaesthesia was maintained with a volatile anaesthetic (desflurane) and remifentanil infusion for analgesia.

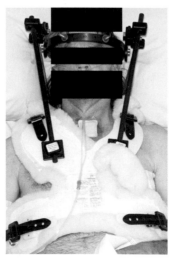

Figure 20.1. A patient with a halo vest *in situ*.

The total surgical time was 6 hours with an uneventful intra-operative course, and blood loss was minimal. The patient was haemodynamically stable throughout the procedure. A halo vest (Figure 20.1) was applied at the end of the procedure.

At the end of the surgery, the volatile agent and the remifentanil infusion were stopped, and the neuromuscular blockade was reversed. Spontaneous ventilation was achieved. The trachea was extubated when the patient was awake, opened his eyes and was obeying commands.

Soon after extubation, the oxygen saturation started to decrease and rapidly reached 90%. The breathing pattern suggested airway obstruction. Bag-mask ventilation following insertion of the oropharyngeal airway failed to ventilate. Suxamethonium was administered, and a size 3 laryngeal mask airway was inserted. Ventilation was suboptimal, but oxygenation was maintained. This continued until the arrival of the ENT surgeon, who performed a tracheostomy. Subsequently, the patient was managed in the critical care unit for a further 24 hours and then transferred to a ward.

The causes for sudden desaturation can be numerous, and they can be different depending on the phase of anaesthesia (Box 20.1)

Box 20.1. Causes for sudden desaturation.

Intra-operatively
- Airway: intraluminal obstruction, displaced airway, secretions, anaphylaxis.
- Breathing: pneumothorax, bronchospasm, underlying chronic lung disease, hypoventilation.
- Circulation: poor peripheral perfusion, pulmonary embolism.
- Exposure: abdominal splinting due to pneumoperitoneum.

At extubation and in the recovery room
- Airway: laryngospasm, obstructed airway.
- Breathing: bronchospasm, pneumothorax, negative pressure pulmonary oedema, aspiration, breath holding, biting on the tube, coughing ++.
- Circulation: myocardial infarction.

Management of a desaturating patient at extubation may depend upon the phase of anaesthesia. A structured way of assessing the patient would be to use the A–E approach, incorporating early administration of 100% oxygen (Box 20.2). If a cause has been identified, treat it as you work your way through the algorithm.

Box 20.2. Algorithm to identify and manage hypoxia at extubation and immediate recovery period.

Airway
- Ensure the patient has a patent airway.
- Consider suctioning of the airway to check patency.
- Assess for any additional noises on inspiration/expiration. Use simple airway manoeuvres to open the airway, or consider the use of adjuncts.

Breathing
- Apply FiO_2 100%.
- Look at the $ETCO_2$ trace if present; any evidence of an obstructive pattern.
- Inspection of chest wall movements: 'seesaw' breathing pattern.
- Palpation of the chest wall: ensure bilateral equal chest wall movements.
- Percussion of the chest wall: looking for hyperresonance suggestive of a pneumothorax, or hyperresonance suggestive of collapse/consolidation.
- Auscultate the chest: assess for wheeze, fine crackles suggestive of pulmonary oedema, and coarse crackles suggestive of consolidation.

Circulation
- Assess peripheral perfusion: consider administration of fluid bolus/vasopressor support. If there is persistent hypoxia: consider an increase in dead space as an example of pulmonary embolism.

Disability
- Consider deepening anaesthesia or inducing anaesthesia and neuromuscular blockade.
- Consider front-of-neck access if the 'cannot ventilate and cannot oxygenate' situation arises.

How would you manage this case differently?

- This patient is likely to have developed airway obstruction, possibly due to retropharyngeal oedema or haematoma from a spinal injury. A careful airway evaluation is essential before extubation.
- Tracheal extubation is a high-risk phase of anaesthesia. Extubation is an elective procedure and careful planning is important. An example of an extubation guideline to aid decision making is shown in Figure 20.2.

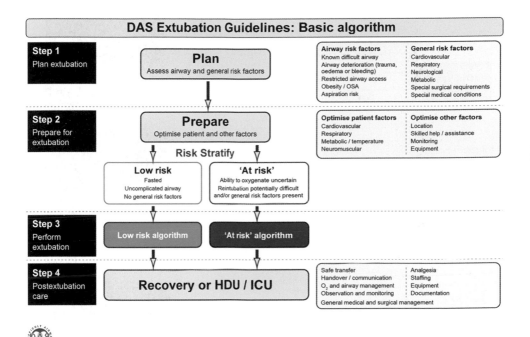

Figure 20.2. Difficult Airway Society extubation guidelines: basic algorithm. *Reproduced with permission from the Difficult Airway Society, © 2011.*

- DAS 'at-risk' extubation guidelines (Figure 20.3) describe three different advanced techniques of extubation. These include the use of remifentanil, the exchange of the tracheal tube for a supraglottic airway device and the use of an airway exchange catheter.

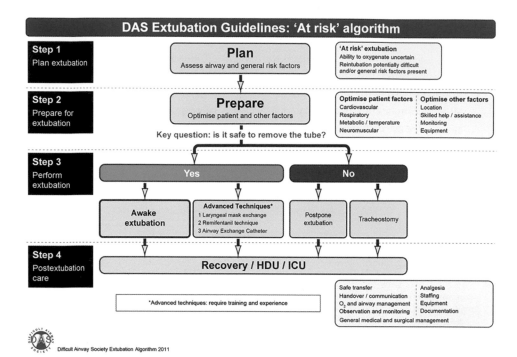

Figure 20.3. Difficult Airway Society extubation guidelines: at-risk algorithm. *Reproduced with permission from the Difficult Airway Society, © 2011.*

- Due to halo vest fixation and immobilisation of the cervical spine, airway access, laryngoscopy and tracheal intubation are anticipated to be difficult in this patient.
- The use of an airway exchange catheter allows reintubation by 'railroading' the tracheal tube over the exchange catheter.
- Another option is to postpone extubation. If there is a potential for airway deterioration at the end of the surgery, delaying extubation and a period of ventilation in the intensive care unit would allow airway oedema to settle, and extubation can be performed following detailed airway evaluation.
- An elective tracheostomy can be considered for situations in which airway deterioration is likely to persist for a longer period or in the presence of risk factors for respiratory failure.
- A clear extubation plan should be communicated to the team, including plans for reintubation if required.

Why can extubation be dangerous?

Airway problems are common during the emergence and recovery phase of anaesthesia. The 4th National Audit Project of the Royal College of Anaesthetists and Difficult Airway Society identified 133 reports of major airway complications at emergence or in the recovery period. In all reported cases, airway obstruction was the root cause.

Extubation is a dynamic phase of anaesthesia that can lead to many systemic causes of instability, as shown in Box 20.3. Specific concerns during extubation are reviewed in Case scenario 21.

Box 20.3. Causes of systemic instability at the point of extubation.

Airway irritation
- Coughing/bucking.
- Laryngospasm.
- Bronchospasm.

Obtunded reflexes
- Aspiration risk.
- Breath holding.
- Biting, leading to damage to the endotracheal tube, leading to a leak if perforated or obstruction if a reinforced tube.

Cardiovascular changes
- Hypertension.
- Arrhythmias.
- Risk of myocardial ischaemia.
- Raised intracranial and intraocular pressures.

Trauma
- Dental damage.
- Airway oedema.

Drug effects
- Residual neuromuscular blockade.

- With a thick pad of fat on the front of the neck, it was impossible to palpate the cricothyroid membrane.

Further examination of the range of neck movements was not attempted due to the nature of the illness.

Investigations

An urgent MRI scan of the spine was performed and showed severe cervical and thoracic canal stenosis with compression of the cervical spinal cord (Figure 21.1).

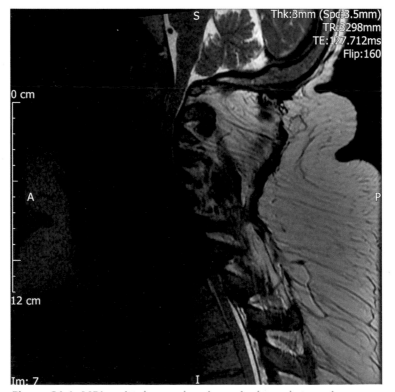

Figure 21.1. MRI sagittal scan showing spinal canal stenosis.

Based on these findings, the neurosurgical team arranged an urgent surgical decompression of the spinal cord from the C4 to the T2 level and lateral mass fixation of the spine and a T7 to T9 laminectomy.

How this case was managed

Pre-operative management

The likelihood of difficult tracheal intubation in this patient was high. Added to that was the distinct possibility of difficult insertion of a supraglottic airway device, difficult face mask ventilation and a difficult cricothyroidotomy.

The anaesthetist made preparations for an awake oral fibreoptic intubation. The airway was anaesthetised with a topical application of 4% lidocaine solution. A carefully titrated target-controlled infusion of remifentanil was used for conscious sedation.

After adequate anaesthesia of the airway and a level of sedation were achieved, the fibreoptic bronchoscope was easily passed into the trachea. A 7.5mm ID reinforced tracheal tube was then passed over the bronchoscope, but an obstruction was encountered at the level of the larynx and the tube could not be 'railroaded' past the vocal cords. Most probably, the tube tip was impinging at the arytenoids (as shown in Figure 11.5A). The quality of airway anaesthesia achieved was excellent, and the patient did not report discomfort during the passage of the bronchoscope or the endotracheal tube. Therefore, a second attempt at intubation was undertaken with the use of a smaller, 7mm ID tracheal tube. Again, an obstruction to the passage of the tube was encountered and the procedure had to be abandoned.

What was the next attempt at securing the airway in this situation?

The anaesthetist made a third attempt at awake fibreoptic intubation. This time a 6mm tube was used, and the trachea was successfully intubated.

The surgery was technically difficult, took 10 hours to complete and finished at 10 p.m. The blood loss was estimated at 1500ml. The patient received an allogeneic blood transfusion and was haemodynamically stable at the end of the procedure. An arterial blood gas sample showed adequate oxygenation and no significant metabolic disturbances.

What was the plan for extubation?

The anaesthetist judged the risk of postoperative respiratory insufficiency in this patient to be high, with risk factors including morbid obesity, the possibility of osteodystrophy-related decreased muscle mass and a long operating time in a prone position. Considering the initial difficulties with tracheal intubation, as well as reduced staffing levels due to the late finishing time, tracheal extubation was postponed until the daytime hours. Tracheal extubation is an elective procedure. Therefore, it should be well planned

---

Box 21.1. Various factors that may lead to problems at extubation.

- Exaggerated reflexes.
- Obtunded reflexes.
- Obesity.
- Obstructive sleep apnoea.
- Residual neuromuscular blockade.
- Depletion of oxygen store.
- Airway injury.
- Surgical/anaesthetic interventions.
- Physiological compromise in other systems.
- Human factor-related issues (equipment and staffing).

(Figures 20.2 and 20.3). Examples of various factors that may lead to problems at extubation are summarised in Box 21.1.

The patient was transferred to the intensive care unit, and tracheal extubation was performed the next morning. As this was an at-risk extubation, a guidewire from a staged extubation set (Figure 21.2) was inserted through the tube into the trachea before extubation. The guidewire was left *in situ* (Figure 21.3) and remained well tolerated by the patient until it was removed 24 hours later.

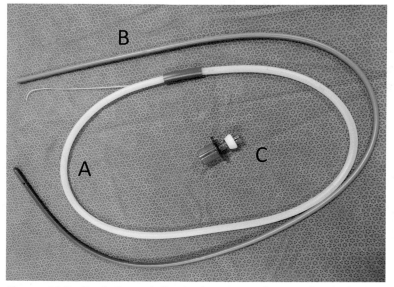

Figure 21.2. Cook Staged Extubation Set. A) Staged extubation guidewire. B) Staged reintubation catheter. C) Rapi-Fit® adapter.

The staged extubation set allows a safe method to reintubate the patient if extubation fails. The kit contains a soft-tipped wire that is well tolerated *in situ* by awake patients. There is a reintubation catheter that can be used to deliver oxygen with the use of the Rapi-Fit® adapter and acts as a bougie/airway exchange catheter to allow a tracheal tube to be 'railroaded' into position.

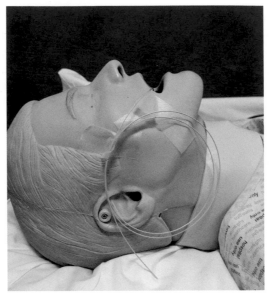

Figure 21.3. Guidewire from the staged extubation kit secured to the face.

If reintubation is required:

- Pass the staged reintubation catheter over the guidewire into the trachea.
- 'Railroad' the tracheal tube over the catheter.
- Remove the guidewire and catheter and confirm the correct placement of the tracheal tube with capnography.

How would you manage this case differently?

- A combination videolaryngoscope and fibreoptic scope could have improved the success rate. Visualisation of tube impingement using a hyperangulated videolaryngoscope will allow manipulation of the tracheal tube under vision. Anticlockwise rotation is the manoeuvre used most commonly to facilitate the passage of the tube through the cords.

- This patient had anticipated difficulty in face mask ventilation, supraglottic airway insertion, tracheal intubation and front-of-neck access. In a situation during awake tracheal intubation, if worsening airway obstruction develops, then emergency front-of-neck access needs to be performed. However, in this patient, emergency front-of-neck access would be challenging. Therefore, a well planned airway management strategy is essential. Additional help should be arranged early, especially for an anaesthetist with experience in difficult airway management.
- Impingement of the tracheal tube at the arytenoids is a recognised problem. The larger the tube size in relation to the size of the fibreoptic scope, the higher the chances of tube impingement. The various solutions include the insertion of a smaller sized tube between the fibreoptic scope and a larger tube and using a tracheal tube with a shorter bevel, such as an intubating LMA tube (Figure 11.6).
- A possible solution includes using a smaller size tube or a larger 5.5mm fibrescope to allow easy 'railroading' of a tracheal tube.
- Preloading the tube with the bevel facing backward minimises the impingement at the arytenoids and facilitates the 'railroading' of the tube over the fibreoptic scope (Figure 21.4).
- Calling for help from a second anaesthetist with experience in managing difficult airways may have helped with troubleshooting the cause of the problem. Preparations should also be made for emergency front-of-neck access if complete airway obstruction develops. In the above case, due to the short neck and impalpable cricothyroid membrane, it would be extremely challenging. It is good practice to scan the front of the neck using ultrasound and mark the cricothyroid membrane and tracheal rings.
- Difficulties may arise at any stage of awake tracheal intubation that may lead to complications. These are listed in Figure 21.5. In this case, there were difficulties encountered at the level of the vocal cords.

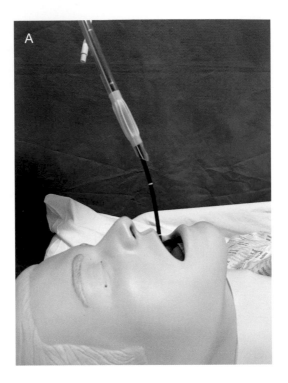

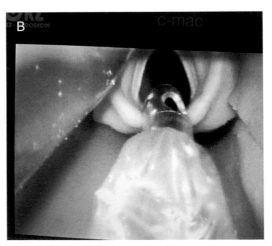

Figure 21.4. A) Tube preloaded on the scope with the bevel faced backwards (posteriorly). B) Tube bevel entering the glottis.

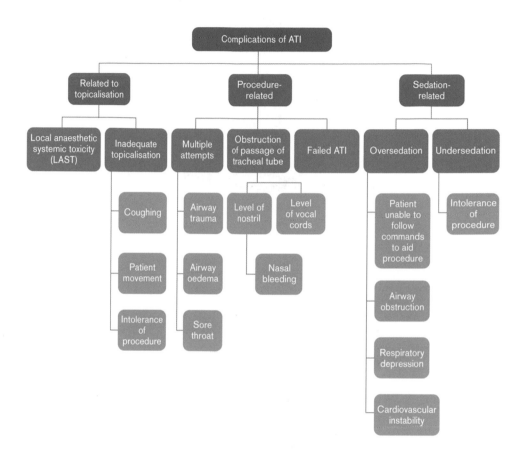

Figure 21.5. Complications of awake tracheal intubation.

What potential complications are there with awake tracheal intubations (ATI)?

- The use of checklists (Table 21.1) and cognitive aids are useful in troubleshooting problems occurring during awake tracheal intubation.

Table 21.1. An example of a checklist for awake tracheal intubation.	
Patient preparation	Assessment of the patient: provide a detailed explanation and obtain consent; provide a patient leaflet on awake intubation; oxygenation, consider high-flow nasal oxygen; reliable IV access; optimum patient position; locate cricothyroid membrane; consider conscious sedation; allocate roles — operator (endoscopist), monitoring the patient, administration of drugs.
Equipment and drugs	Monitoring equipment: optimum ergonomics; correct size fibreoptic scope and tracheal tube; equipment for topicalisation of local anaesthetic; calculate the maximum dose based on lean body weight; syringe pumps and sedative drugs; plan for induction and maintenance of anaesthesia.
Preparation for failure	What if the awake intubation fails; would you postpone the procedure? Is a second anaesthetist required? Is an ENT surgeon available? Communicate the plan with the team.
Performing the procedure	Check topicalisation; check sedation level; perform endoscopy; confirm correct placement of the tube.

Key points

- Although awake tracheal intubation remains the most suitable option for the management of anticipated difficult intubations, complications and failure may occur.
- Measures for troubleshooting during the procedure should be planned. Adequate preparation minimises the risk of failure.
- In a situation where awake fibreoptic intubation fails, if the patient is stable, a mini-team brief should be performed, and available options, including postponing the procedure, should be considered.

References

1. Asai T, Shingu K. Difficulty in advancing a tracheal tube over a fibreoptic bronchoscope: incidence, causes and solutions. *Br J Anaesth* 2004; 92(6): 870-81.

2. Biro P, Priebe HJ. Staged extubation strategy: is an airway exchange catheter the answer? *Anesth Analg* 2007; 105(5): 1182-5.

3. Difficult Airway Society Extubation Guidelines Group, Popat M, Mitchell V, *et al.* Difficult Airway Society guidelines for the management of tracheal extubation. *Anaesthesia* 2012; 67(3): 318-40.

4. Duggan LV, Law JA, Murphy MF. Brief review: supplementing oxygen through an airway exchange catheter: efficacy, complications, and recommendations. *Can J Anaesth* 2011; 58(6): 560-8.

5. Grange K, Mushambi MC, Jaladi S, Athanassoglou V. Techniques and complications of awake fibre-optic intubation – a survey of Difficult Airway Society members. *Trends Anaesth Crit Care* 2019; 28: 21-6.

6. Marfin AG, Iqbal R, Mihm F, *et al.* Determination of the site of tracheal tube impingement during nasotracheal fibreoptic intubation. *Anaesthesia* 2006; 61(7): 646-50.

7. Mort TC. Continuous airway access for the difficult extubation: the efficacy of the airway exchange catheter. *Anesth Analg* 2007; 105(5): 1357-62.

8. Vora J, Leslie D, Stacey M. Awake tracheal intubation. *BJA Educ* 2022; 22(8): 298-305.

Case scenario 22

Introduction

A 65-year-old man has been an inpatient in an ENT ward for 3 weeks following a hemi-mandibulectomy and a reconstruction of the tissue defect with a free fibula flap. The surgery was uneventful, and a tracheostomy was performed at the time of the procedure.

The free tissue transfer was successful but, unfortunately, the patient developed a haematoma at the donor site of the graft. The wound was evacuated under general anaesthesia a week after the initial surgery.

In the following days, the site of the mandibulectomy continued to heal well and the tracheostomy was decannulated.

The patient remained in hospital, as he required ongoing care of his leg wound. Three weeks after the initial operation, he presented for examination and primary closure of the leg wound under general anaesthesia.

Past medical history

He had no other past medical history to note.

Clinical examination

The anaesthetist reviewed the patient on the ward and performed a pre-operative assessment. It was noted that the tracheostomy had been decannulated 5 days before. The patient's hemi-mandibulectomy wound had healed by this time.

An airway examination revealed the following:

- An inter-incisor gap of 3.5cm.
- Normal neck flexion and extension.
- Mallampati score of 3.

A review of the anaesthetic chart from his last operation showed anaesthesia was induced and maintained using an inhalational technique via the tracheostomy tube when presented for the evacuation of haematoma at the leg wound, a week after the surgery. The induction of anaesthesia, and the intra-operative and postoperative course were uneventful.

Investigations

Postoperative routine investigations were within the normal range.

How this case was managed

Because of the recent, complex maxillofacial procedure, the anaesthetist decided to perform awake fibreoptic intubation and discussed this plan with the patient.

However, once the patient arrived at the anaesthetic room, the anaesthetist changed the intubation plan. He now decided to perform an intravenous induction of anaesthesia with maintenance of the airway via an i-gel® supraglottic airway device.

General anaesthesia was induced with fentanyl and propofol. When the insertion of an i-gel® was attempted, the anaesthetist encountered difficulties in inserting the device. Following the insertion of an i-gel®, ventilation through the device was ineffective, leading to desaturation of the patient.

How this situation was managed

The i-gel® was removed. Face mask ventilation was commenced but also proved to be difficult. The maxillofacial surgeon was called in urgently and inserted a tracheostomy tube via the previous tracheostomy site.

The anaesthetist, a consultant with years of experience in airway management, was unable to explain why he decided to radically change the previously formulated airway management plan. It is a decision-making dilemma in which the human brain accepts management options that are easy and quick to perform. This can then turn out to be a high-risk strategy.

How would you manage this case differently?

- With a history of previous maxillofacial surgery, there was a risk that a supraglottic airway device may not sit well due to anatomical changes. Even in patients with normal anatomy, in 50–80% of cases, supraglottic airway devices have been shown to be malpositioned in imaging studies. The epiglottis has been shown to sit within the bowl of the laryngeal mask in 50% of patients when evaluated using a fibreoptic device post-insertion. When correctly placed, the tip of the supraglottic airway device rests against the upper oesophageal sphincter (Figure 22.1).
- In this case, an initial safe anaesthetic plan was in place based on accurate patient information. It is important to draft an airway management plan based on the airway assessment and available clinical information. In addition to a primary plan, additional plans should be in place to manage any failure. This airway management strategy should be verbalised to the theatre team and strictly adhered to. In this case, the safest plan would have been to perform an awake nasal fibreoptic intubation. If there were no contraindications, regional anaesthesia could also have been considered.
- The 4th National Audit Project of the Royal College of Anaesthetists (NAP4) examined major complications in airway management and concluded that human factors could have contributed to 40% of the cases reported. Table 22.1 shows common human factors that can affect the management of airway emergencies.

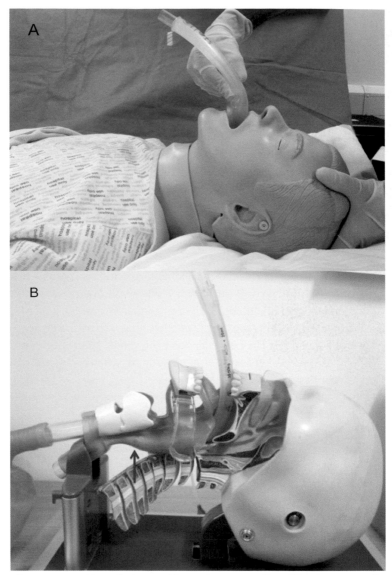

Figure 22.1. A) Technique of inserting a SAD (i-gel®). B) A correctly positioned LMA with the tip (arrow) resting against the upper oesophageal sphincter.

Table 22.1. Human factors in airway emergencies.

Human factors category	Subtypes	Examples
Individual	Situational awareness	Attention and vigilance, perception, memory
	Decision making	Poor judgement, failure to re-evaluate
	Personality	Overconfidence, pride, guilt
	Technical	Inadequate skill, inadequate pre-operative assessment
	Performance-shaping factors	Stress, fatigue, hunger
Team	Situational awareness	Attention and vigilance, perception, memory
	Behavioural	Communication, poor teamwork/coordination
	Social	Conflict, awkwardness
	Workplace	Poor time management, limitations in strategies
Environmental	Equipment	Clutter, equipment faults, inconsistent storage
	Workspace	Crowding, poor ergonomics
	Ambience	Inadequate lighting, noise
Organisational	Policies/procedures	Lack of incident reporting, no morbidity/mortality meetings
	Culture	Management team, perceived norms, patient safety
	Job factors	Task complexity, overload, poor staffing levels
	Training/supervision	Lack of training, poor supervision

Why do serious airway complications occur?

- Lack of knowledge of airway assessment and management. There is no single reliable tool to accurately predict and quantify the difficulty in airway management.
- Lack of confidence in the procedural skill (for example, awake fibreoptic intubation) encourages the operator to omit the procedure from the management strategy.
- Persistent attempts at a single option, lack of situational awareness, and not considering alternative options increase airway morbidity and mortality.
- The attitude of the operator may encourage them to ignore the clinical findings and to use a high-risk strategy.

What factors may cause someone to change their initial airway management plan?

It is not clear what made the anaesthetist change his initial plan. Within this case, we could look at the mental model used by the anaesthetist to make sense of the scenario. A mental model is a psychological representation

---

Box 22.1. Examples of mental models.

- Circle of competence: providing a way to compare what we know versus what we think we know.
- First principles thinking: in which a problem is identified that is then deconstructed before a solution is found.
- Model of compounding: used predominantly in the financial world. It describes how interest added to a fixed sum gains further interest. For example, someone who exercises regularly from an early age will be healthier and more mobile in older age.
- The map is not the territory: maps represent a snapshot of time and may not be a perfect representation of reality.

of a real, hypothetical or imaginary situation. It is an explanation of a person's thought process or what they expect to happen. Box 22.1 gives examples of different mental models that professionals use to organise their thinking.

Key points

- Due to the recent history of maxillofacial surgery, a high level of vigilance should be maintained as more difficult intubation, and complications associated with intubation (such as bleeding), may be higher.
- Careful attention to human factors is crucial when dealing with a patient with a potentially difficult airway. The most common factors affecting airway management decisions include situational awareness, job factors and performance-shaping factors.
- Asking yourself questions about limitations, probable complications, possible causes for deterioration, the likelihood of success, and the potential pitfalls may help to clarify the mental model that should be used.

References

1. Cook TM, Woodall N, Frerk C; 4th National Audit Project. Major complications of airway management in the UK: results of the 4th National Audit Project of the Royal College of Anaesthetists and the Difficult Airway Society. Part 1: anaesthesia. *Br J Anaesth* 2011; 106(5): 617-31.

2. Gleeson S, Groom P, Mercer S. Human factors in complex airway management. *BJA Educ* 2016; 16(6): 191-7.

3. Rewers M, Chrimes N. Human factors in airway management. In: Cook T, Kristensen SM, Eds. *Core Topics in Airway Management*. Cambridge University Press; 2020.

4. Thondebavi M. Mental models and the anaesthetist. *J Anaesth Crit Care Case Rep* 2018; 4(3): 7-8.

5. Van Zundert AA, Kumar CM, Van Zundert TC. Malpositioning of supraglottic airway devices: preventive and corrective strategies. *Br J Anaesth* 2016; 116(5): 579-82.

Case scenario 23

Introduction

A 1.8kg 35-week-old twin neonate presented to the emergency department. A pre-hospital paediatric medical alert had been activated by the ambulance crew conveying the infant due to an episode of apnoea during transfer.

Past medical history

She was born at 30 weeks with her twin via emergency Caesarean section for foetal distress. She spent 4 weeks in neonatal intensive care due to prematurity and was discharged home well.

Clinical examination

Upon arrival at the hospital, she required some breaths via the T-piece breathing circuit, after which she resumed spontaneous breathing effort.

Two hours after arrival in the emergency department, a paediatric emergency call was activated for the same child due to a further apnoea spell from which she was slow to recover. The child required bag-mask ventilation with 100% oxygen. Oxygen saturations were maintained at 98%. As spontaneous efforts were minimal and there was an increased frequency of apnoea episodes, a decision was made to continue to intubation and ventilation.

The paediatric medical team had made a provisional diagnosis of bronchiolitis. Therefore, the child was transferred to the paediatric high dependency unit (HDU) for monitoring.

Investigations

- Full bloods were taken, with the results still pending.
- CXR was normal.

What would be your concerns with this case?

- Ex-premature infant — corrected age 35 weeks.
- Low body weight requiring dose adjustments.
- Urgent need for intubation and ventilation due to presentation — time pressure.
- Human factors — personal experience of intubating such a small infant.
- Risk of airway oedema with recurrent airway manipulation.
- Risk of diaphragmatic splinting due to gas build-up in the stomach during bag-mask ventilation causing impaired ventilation.

How this case was managed

To prepare for tracheal intubation, roles were allocated to each of the team members for each of the key tasks, including team leadership, airway, scribing and monitoring the patients. An experienced operating department practitioner (anaesthetic assistant) was also present as part of the team. They were asked to prepare the paediatric airway equipment and provide airway assistance during the intubation attempt.

Given the extreme age and size of the child, a paediatric specialist anaesthetist was requested to attend and be the '1st intubator'. A neonatal specialist registrar was also present as part of the team, and they were asked to be the '2nd intubator'.

The infant was given 2mg/kg ketamine (3.6mg) and 1mg/kg rocuronium (1.8mg) to induce anaesthesia and provide neuromuscular blockade. Gentle manual ventilation was provided using the T-piece. Laryngoscopy was performed using a GlideScope® videolaryngoscope (VL) and a Miller size 0

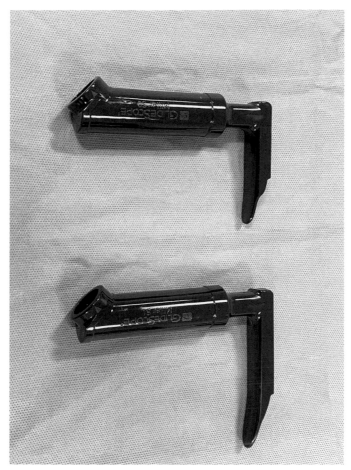

Figure 23.1. Miller blades.

blade (Figure 23.1); only part of the glottic opening was visible on the VL screen or directly. A size 3 cuffed oral endotracheal tube was passed through the vocal cords. Chest rise, misting and end-tidal CO_2 ($EtCO_2$) were obtained. However, the $EtCO_2$ trace was lost after four breaths, so the endotracheal tube was removed and returned to manual mask ventilation. There was a brief desaturation that self-corrected.

What was the next step?

Following discussion amongst the team, it was decided to have a further attempt with the neonatal registrar taking the lead, given their more regular experience with neonatal intubation. A standard direct Miller laryngoscope was used for the second attempt. Again, a limited view was obtained, and a size 3 cuffed oral tracheal tube could be passed through the vocal cords. Again, EtCO$_2$ was achieved but rapidly tailed off and was removed. The neonatal registrar had one further attempt but with the same result.

It was becoming increasingly difficult to ventilate via the mask and T-piece, so a size 1 i-gel® was placed and ventilation continued. Given the difficulty with intubation, a discussion was held between team members to decide the next step. Additional help was called for from the on-call consultant neonatologist. Upon their arrival, two further attempts at intubation were carried out, ensuring further boluses of sedation and muscle relaxant were given.

Unfortunately, these further attempts were also unsuccessful, so oxygenation was maintained using the i-gel®. An intravenous morphine infusion was commenced for sedation as per local protocols.

During the intubation attempts, discussions were had with the regional paediatric critical care advice and transfer service. Given the need for the intubation, the patient would need to be moved to a separate level 3 paediatric critical care facility, as the local hospital could only support level 2. Given the difficulty in intubation, a direct conversation was had between the anaesthetist, the patient's family and the paediatric critical care consultant. The retrieval team was dispatched, with the consultant following in a separate vehicle.

With the paediatric critical care team present, the trachea was successfully intubated using a paediatric fibreoptic scope. Once the airway was secured, the patient was transferred to the regional children's hospital where ear, nose and throat (ENT) surgeons were waiting.

How would you manage this case differently?

- The case reflects the unusual situation of an unanticipated difficult airway in a neonate. At present, there are no Difficult Airway Society (DAS) guidelines for neonates. The DAS has guidance covering management of the unanticipated difficult airway from a 1-year-old or older. The British Association of Perinatal Medicine (BAPM) has

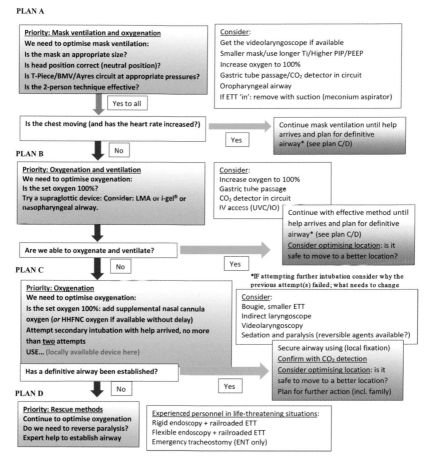

Figure 23.2. BAPM difficult airway algorithm. *Reproduced with permission from the BAPM. © BAPM, 2020. https://www.bapm.org/resources/199-managing-the-difficult-airway-in-the-neonate. Continued overleaf.*

Appendix 1 – BAPM Framework algorithm

Unexpected Difficult Airway (Neonates)
Read all the text in **BOLD** aloud to the team:
VERBALISE AS CHALLENGE AND RESPONSE.
Yes/No responses required from team leader

Immediate actions**: We have a difficult airway situation**

1. Has someone called for expert help? Send a specific team member to call for help (numbers below):

Tell them to state: 'We have a difficult airway situation in (state your location). Please attend immediately.'

- 1)..
- 2)..
- 3)..

2. Has the difficult airway box been located and retrieved?

If not: retrieve and open the difficult airway box, located at:

....

NOW TURN OVER THIS SHEET AND READ FROM 'PLAN A'

Other information:

Medication for sedation/paralysis: Type/dose...

Medication for reversal of sedation/paralysis: Type/dose...............................

Location of specific equipment (e.g. ENT scopes, tracheostomy kit)

(what)............................... (where)..

....

To be accessed by contacting ....

on ....

Figure 23.2. BAPM difficult airway algorithm. *Reproduced with permission from the BAPM. © BAPM, 2020. https://www.bapm.org/resources/199-managing-the-difficult-airway-in-the-neonate. Continued overleaf.*

Appendix 2: Equipment: visual inventory

Store with difficult airway box

PLAN A Name and location of equipment	Add photographs here
PLAN B Name and location of equipment	Add photographs here
PLAN C Name and location of equipment	Add photographs here
PLAN D Name and location of equipment	Add photographs here

Figure 23.2. BAPM difficult airway algorithm. *Reproduced with permission from the BAPM. © BAPM, 2020. https://www.bapm.org/resources/199-managing-the-difficult-airway-in-the-neonate.*

published guidelines (see References) which follow a similar Plan A to Plan C management plan and prioritise oxygenation at every step.

- The paediatric fibrescope should be kept in a location known to members of staff and easily accessible in such times as per difficult intubation algorithms (Figure 23.2).
- The importance of a 'stop' moment is reflected upon to reassess the approach required to manage the human factors evident in this scenario. Communication with the tertiary centre could have been opened earlier to prevent excessive manipulation of the paediatric airway. This would reduce the risk of total airway obstruction due to oedema.

How would you approach difficult neonatal intubation?

In the case described above, there were five attempts at intubation. The number of attempts in a difficult airway scenario can be challenging. The relevant DAS guidance would suggest three attempts, with one further attempt by an experienced intubator. Whilst the approach is valid, the particular circumstances must be taken into account, including the stability of the patient, the availability of equipment that may help and the technical skills of the team members. In this case, two of the three different intubators were consultants. After failure of both the consultant anaesthetist and the neonatal registrar (three of the five attempts), the neonatal consultant had two further attempts. The key is the recognition that the airway is difficult and to maintain oxygenation. In this case, the airway was becoming increasingly difficult to maintain even with a mask and supraglottic devices, probably due to airway swelling and oedema. Once this has been recognised, as in this case, it was important to stop further attempts and continue discussions with the tertiary centre. Due to concerns of airway swelling, intravenous dexamethasone was given early, as further intervention later in this child's treatment was likely to be necessary.

Of note, in this case, was the need for transfer. The presenting hospital only had facilities for level 2 paediatric critical care, not level 3, necessitating an inter-hospital transfer. This added some complexity to the airway management, as securing the airway during transfer has additional logistical and human factor concerns in addition to those already described above. As such, securing the airway before the transfer was important. The current

Intensive Care Society guidelines concerning the transfer of a critically ill patient do not specify the type of airway device that could be used to facilitate the transfer. In this case, there may have been an argument for transferring the child using a well secured i-gel® (supraglottic airway device) as long as oxygenation and gas exchange were adequate. This would allow transfer to a centre with experienced paediatric ENT and anaesthetic clinicians if considered adequate. However, there are inherent risks in carrying out a transfer in this way and would be a risk-benefit decision, as options would be limited should the supraglottic airway device become dislodged en route.

How would you manage the team dynamics through this scenario?

Situations that involve an unanticipated difficult airway are inherently stressful, both to the individual and to the wider team. This being a paediatric case only adds to heighten this level of stress. There is strong evidence that a clear team leader and clear role allocations can help a team work well together to manage clinical situations that, in themselves, help to manage the stress and anxiety incumbent with it. In this scenario, a clear team leader was identified and roles were clearly allocated with the plan discussed before the intubation attempt. This had the advantage that, when problems were faced, the team was ready and well versed, whilst achieving the best result for the patient. In addition to this, clear lines of communication were maintained between the clinical team directly managing the child and the paediatric retrieval team, so that they were aware of the case and could mobilise resources promptly and effectively.

Key points

- Neonatal difficult airway management may require using different resources and different team members for paediatric and adult difficult intubations. They may need to be contacted early, as they may only be on site during normal working hours.
- Managing the team and maintaining good communication are imperative to safe airway management for the neonate.

References

1. British Association of Perinatal Medicine. Managing the Difficult Airway in the Neonate; A BAPM Framework for Practice. 2020. Available from: https://www.bapm.org/resources/199-managing-the-difficult-airway-in-the-neonate.

2. Difficult Airway Society. Paediatric Difficult Airway Guidelines 2015. Available from: https://das.uk.com/guidelines/downloads.html.

Index